D1344035

THE
MEANING
OF PAIN

THE
MEANING
OF PAIN

What it is, why we feel it,
and how to overcome it

NICK POTTER

Published in 2019 by
Short Books, Unit 316, ScreenWorks, 22 Highbury Grove,
London, N5 2ER

10 9 8 7 6 5 4 3 2 1

A CIP catalogue record for this book
is available from the British Library.

ISBN: 978-1-78072-390-7

Illustrations by Helena Sutcliffe
Cover design by Two Associates

Printed at CPI Group (UK) Ltd, Croydon, CR0 4YY

To my amazing wife Bex and my two wonderful children Emi and Jack.

'It is not to see something first, but to establish solid connections between the previously known and the hitherto unknown, that constitutes the essence of scientific discovery. It is this process of tying together which can best promote true understanding and real progress.'

Hans Selye, *The Stress of Life*

CONTENTS

INTRODUCTION

'It is far more important to understand what person the
disease has than what disease the person has.'

– Hippocrates

I always like to know why someone decides to write a book
– what drives them to do it and whether they have 'skin in
the game' either professionally or through personal experience. When it comes to pain, I think I have both.

Professionally, I am a consultant osteopath, and during 27 years of clinical practice, hundreds of patients have
entrusted their problems and bodies to me. I now run a
clinic at the Princess Grace Hospital in London, and before
that spent 17 years at the London Spine Clinic, where I
specialised in conditions of the cervical spine, the area
around the neck. I became known there as 'Nick the neck',
and was very proud of my results in reducing neck surgery
by 80 per cent.

After completing my degree in osteopathic medicine
in London, I soon realised that, although university had

given me a wonderful training and I had had some inspirational teachers, it wasn't quite enough. So I went on to do more training, and worked in the US, France, Australia and Germany. Exposed to a wide variety of medical and non-medical approaches in different cultural settings, I gradually built my toolbox of skills.

For the past two decades, my life has been split between my hospital clinic and the world we call performance science, or performance medicine, which focuses on the optimisation of performance, especially in sports. In the late 1990s when the Chelsea Harbour Club opened in London, a team of us set up a sports medicine clinic called Total Health, where we took a multidisciplinary approach to health and fitness which was quite revolutionary for its time. From there I went in 1999 to join the Institut Biomédical Sports et Vie (IBSV), set up by Dr François Duforez, who was doctor to the Formula One driver Alain Prost. Based in Paris, the IBSV (later renamed vielife) carried out driver assessments to improve performance, and as part of this we quickly realised the importance of data and building trends in the less obvious arenas of sleep, stress, global travel, nutrition, light exposure, mindset and so on. What we did not have at the time was Bluetooth and wireless technology to monitor these trends more regularly and accurately – that would prove to be a game changer. But, even without these digital aids, we soon saw that what we were learning about the treatment of elite sportsmen, particularly with regard to stress, could have a much wider application – not least in the corporate world. We started to formulate a special set of assessments for people operating in a high-stress executive environment under the notion of the 'corporate athlete'. And – this being the frenetic early 2000s – before long CEOs and board-level executives who were suffering with issues similar to those that affected elite athletes started coming to us for help. Like top athletes, people at executive level in high-stress companies can easily become isolated from their colleagues and have to bury the stress that they feel in case it shows weakness. This takes its toll and manifests in their physiology, which we had learned to measure. The two most commonly complained of issues were sleep and musculoskeletal pain. Ultimately, both were caused by stress. I am still using this application today – in particular, in recent years, working for a leading hedge fund, where I look at the impact of stress on traders and how to manage it.

That early experience of working in performance medicine – which also included stints with the Jordanian, Jaguar and McLaren Formula One teams, as well as in elite golf, tennis and athletics – gave me a number of things. It indulged my obsession with people-watching as it involved really working out what made humans tick. And it showed me that each and every athlete was different and therefore a general training programme would never suffice. I realise now that we were way ahead of our time and I was phenomenally lucky to work with such ground-breaking experts. It has also been hugely influential in the way I work in a clinical setting.

When I first started in clinical practice, osteopathy was seen by some as very 'alternative' and 'complementary', even shrouded in charlatanism and quackery. Indeed, GPs could be disciplined for referring a patient to one. Oh, how things have changed! Over the years I have seen its principles embraced by the medical community and have helped in some small way in pioneering its 'scientific art' in a traditional and very medical environment. Many of the new imaging and investigatory techniques that have been developed over the last few years have not only supported but indeed proved the principles and efficacy of the osteopathic philosophy and its techniques.

Having said that, I feel very strongly that, in a bid to become 'recognised' by the orthodox community, we as a profession should not lose any of the philosophy that has set us apart from, and given us the edge on, modern drug- and surgery-based medicine. In recent years, I have seen a pendulum-like swing in modern medicine's approach. It has gone from a technology-driven profession of keyhole surgery and clever drugs to one that is now increasingly wary of interventions of any kind, due to the realisation that many of them, with hindsight, do not work or are, in terms of healing, no better than time. To a large extent, the old interventionist model was born from the need to reduce costs in our health system and to find what was efficient in the short term rather than what really worked. It was driven by a consumer-type demand from patients to be cured and the recognition by drug and surgical companies that there was an exciting demand out there to be satisfied. But what they were missing was that the human body relies on systems that do not work in isolation but are intricately linked in a web of myriad connections, within a unique and conscious being. Nowhere is that truer than in the field of pain.

So why did a 20-year-old from a privileged and very traditional background go into such an uncertain profession? Why did I take 'the road less travelled', as Frost put it?

I was educated at an intensely competitive school in North London, where I was taught to be curious, to develop a love of knowledge and always 'kick the tyres' of what we know. The competitive environment and a healthy fear of failure, though exhausting, meant you could never know enough. It is an attitude that has remained with me since and, as my wife will tell you, I am still exhausting. I also strongly suspect that, had the diagnosis been around in those days, I would have been described as having ADHD.

One of the biggest influences on me during my last years at school was suffering a back injury; indeed, it was a factor in my decision to become an osteopath. I was always quite sporty at school, though also quite a chubby chap, until I lost most of my excess weight and turned it into muscle when I was about 16. By that time I was playing a lot of rugby competitively, and during my last year I proudly captained my school's First XV. I played prop in the front row, and being endlessly compressed by around 40 stone of scrumming youth and at an awkward angle was beginning to cause me recurrent episodes of acute low back pain which would incapacitate me. I tried to soldier on, but eventually I was referred to two people who helped me enormously in managing it: a blind and brilliant physiotherapist who had lost his sight in the Blitz, Mr Berry (I would later work with him and be greatly influenced by him), and an osteopath, whose ability to assess me by just watching my movement and palpating my body was extraordinary.

Both grew very concerned at why an 18-year-old was

having these problems and referred me for an X-ray. It showed that I had been carrying a nasty little fracture in two places for some time. I had quite significant disc damage, too, as I would discover later, which did not show up on the X-ray at the time. Many years later, I am structurally healed, and, as long as I keep myself strong, lean and mobile, I am fine. However, I can still get pain. Why? That is the very important question I will attempt to answer, among a number of others, in this book.

By the way, I mention being large as a kid because it, too, has been formative in my approach to life and my work. I hated being fat, but I loved food more and I became hardened to any unkind teasing I faced. My usual response was to thump the individual concerned, as I tended to be bigger than them, and that ended that. It is amazing how this sort of mental and emotional hurt remains with you, though.

A few months ago, I was sitting in traffic at some lights near home, just by some playing fields. I looked on as, in the distance, a young sports teacher, probably a gap-year student, chose two captains from a group of 11-year-olds. Watching as the two smug-looking favourites picked their teams, one boy by one, I felt a tightening in my chest and a tensioning in my jaw. In my mind's eye, I was transported straight back to my school days, and being one of those waiting to be picked and being seized with dread as the number waned and I knew I would be left standing – 'fatty' me with Josh aka 'specky-skinny-four-eyes' standing next to me. The ignominy of being the last every time was very painful. And here I was, 40 years later, with the nauseating fear of failure still there. In fact, I was so struck by this emotion, that I was seized by the need to explain to the coach the effect of his technique on the two boys inevitably left to last. So I parked up, jogged over and did exactly that.

Expecting to be told to 'bog-off', I was pleasantly surprised when my suggestion was met with grateful interest. The young man was in teacher training and the effect of his actions had not dawned on him. I think he also realised the depth of my ingrained emotion – which was such that I had interrupted my day, parked my car illegally and jogged all the way along the field perimeter to make my point. I simply suggested to him that by making the minimal extra effort of splitting the group in half himself – doing his best to make the sides of roughly equal strength by eye, and making small adjustments where necessary – he would save many kids in the future the misery of being the one who didn't quite make the athletic grade or the social group.

I ambled back to my car, ruminating on what I had just done and feeling faintly satisfied, but also realising that, as if from nowhere, my low back had begun to ache. As I have said, I have carried a back injury all my life. But it has been better for years as I maintain it and know its little ways. And it dawned on me then that I was experiencing what so many people world-wide suffer from every day – and what many of my own patients are afflicted with – the raw physical manifestation of emotional pain. My mind had found the weak spot in my body, the place where the injury had previously existed, to give me a little reminder of past feelings that I had parked. The memory of my playground dread had allowed the physical pain memory to pop up its head; and, as physical pain is easier to salve, it is often substituted for the emotional one.

I made myself take a long, deep breath, which I realised I was holding, and bent down to touch my toes to confirm to myself that all was well down there. And, as I walked on, the pain simply faded. The whole experience gently reminded me of two things: that emotional pain is etched onto our psyches in a way that physical pain rarely is; and that we are each of us products of our environments and our early experiences, which set the tone for all our future behaviour. Pain is not like a disease, something extrinsic to be fought or warded off, but something intrinsic and experiential. I am telling this story because I think it explains many of the beliefs I have now about why it is that we hurt; why medicine and science are 'missing the point' in many areas; and why chronic pain has become a new epidemic, for which we don't yet have the answers.

In this book, I will elaborate on these ideas, and discuss pain in all its guises: what it is, why we feel it and what it means – why pain is at the heart of what it is to be human. I will also look at the relationship between stress and pain and sow some seeds for contemplation about how we see our symptoms and what we can do to fix ourselves.

CHAPTER 1

WHAT IS PAIN?

'Here sighs and cries and shrieks of lamentation
echoed throughout the starless air of Hell.'
– Dante Alighieri, *The Divine Comedy*

You stub your toe, shut your fingers in a door, wake up
with a bad neck or back after moving heavy furniture –
or, worse, experience a sinister ache that could turn out to
be a symptom of something very frightening indeed. Or
perhaps you develop a pain that moves around your body,
and you have no idea what is causing it. We all fear pain,
believing – even if we don't understand the source – that
it is always the harbinger of bad news. We will do almost
anything to avoid it – take to our beds; avoid activities or
work we previously enjoyed; swallow medication that may
prove addictive; even submit to surgery in the hope that
the short-term intense pain of this will alleviate the longer-
term agony.

But what if everything you thought you knew about
pain and where it came from turned out to be wrong or
only half the truth? What if I told you that your experience

of pain in the present moment might in fact be connected with the very origins of *Homo sapiens* – that it might have evolved as a warning of imminent danger?

Don't worry… I'm not about to suggest that your ankle fracture is all in the mind. It hurts, of course it does. No one is doubting that. But we now know there is a great deal more to the experience of the pain you have than just the broken bone, damaged disc or grazed skin. What I'm talking about is the new – but now well-evidenced – bio-psycho-social model of pain science. In these pages, I will endeavour to explain as clearly as possible this complex concept, to help you reframe how you experience pain and spur you into action to seek new ways of approaching and curing, or at least relieving, it.

It may not always be easy to find the help you need but there are enlightened practitioners out there. Slowly but surely, a community of joined-up specialists, providing new and visionary approaches to tackling pain, is growing. To date, the world of pain treatment has unfortunately been as much a mystery for the medical and scientific community as it has for the sufferer. This has been particularly true over the last 20 years, during which medicine and science have been driven predominantly by the pharmaceutical industries, who have tended to follow a reductionist approach, whittling things down to a molecular and cellular level rather than taking into consideration the multiple factors which are key to our understanding of pain. In most conditions A plus B does not necessarily equal C.

So be kind to yourself, for it is not you who have failed to get better but the system we currently have – the legacy of years of pain mismanagement – that has failed to help and educate you.

THE PHANTOM

If we are going to discuss pain – and especially how to overcome it – then we have to start by identifying what it is. The International Association for the Study of Pain defines it as:

> An unpleasant sensory and emotional experience associated with actual or potential tissue damage, or described in terms of such damage

... which, although rather convoluted, is at least a fairly accurate definition and reflects much of our current understanding, because it highlights some of the curious aspects of pain that we will be covering: that it is both a sensory *and* an emotional experience and that it can be caused by both actual and potential tissue damage. Or, wait for it, even no damage at all. Confused? You won't be, I promise.

One thing is undeniable: pain is unpleasant. It is also essential: an experience put there by evolution and nature to alert us to danger. It's what will make us withdraw our finger from a hot plate, say, before any damage is done. Nature, being the cruel mother she is, doesn't care about our contentment or physical well-being, simply that we succeed reproductively and achieve the survival of our genes. She has no remit to make us happy. And, in this sense, pain is our greatest guardian. Pain, nausea, sadness, fear and anxiety... they are all there to protect us from harm in different ways. If we accept them as a necessary part of living, our fear of them should in some way be salved.

But what about the more challenging fact that there needs to be no physical harm or injury for pain to exist? That you can experience severe, even disabling, pain without discernible disease or structural injury? Good examples of this are back pain, migraine, fibromyalgia, chronic fatigue syndrome and ME, all of which I will cover in more detail later on, with some helpful pointers for patients. Each of these conditions causes a great deal of suffering; the symptoms appear from nowhere and incapacitate the sufferer, and yet nothing shows up in blood tests or scans.

And, if that wasn't mind-boggling enough, there are many well-documented cases of individuals who have suffered major injury but report no pain at all; for example, a Second World War veteran who had a chest X-ray which revealed that a bullet had been sitting in his chest for 60 years – with no ill effect.

Before I go any further, let's be very clear. Your pain is real; it hurts; and the symptoms associated with it, such as fatigue and anxiety, are also real. We clinicians have to remember that a patient is always in exactly as much pain as they say they are, and that pain does not have to come from a tangible source to be a valid problem.

How else could we explain Couvade syndrome, a condition in which men have been known to physically experience some of their expectant partners' symptoms, including labour pains? Pain can be a shared phenomenon (more on this later).

What I am about to explain is going to require some processing and mental leaps, but if I do my job right, it will change your whole mindset towards your pain, forever. Knowledge and insight have the power to transform, and in my clinical experience I have found that insight can often be more helpful to people than advice. As the palliative care and addiction expert Dr Gabor Maté says: 'If we gain the ability to look into ourselves with honesty, compassion and with unclouded vision we can identify the ways in which we need to take care of ourselves.'[1]

Frustratingly for me and my practitioner colleagues in the fight against pain, there are very few good descriptive words in the English language to describe the concept of pain and its elements. This is partly because all of the sensory processes that occur in the body and brain, which combine to produce pain, occur at an unconscious or subconscious level. Yes, that's right: it is only when the subconscious brain decides that the information it is getting is important enough that it makes us consciously aware of it so that we experience it as pain. In fact, most of the time pain is the conscious manifestation of a multitude of responses and processes which occur at a neuro-psychological level.

However, say anything that contains the word 'psychological' to a patient and you risk being misconstrued as insinuating that their pain is 'all in the head' or, worse, that they are neurotic or wimpy or simply bonkers – whereas nothing could be further from the truth.

Another reason we are so ill-equipped to explain pain is that our current understanding of it is but a few years old. Until recently, medicine operated in a Cartesian world. René Descartes (1596–1650) was the *Cogito ergo sum* (I think therefore I am) guy, a French philosopher who wrote extensively on consciousness and existence and had a profound influence on the philosophy of healthcare and medicine. He was among the first to introduce the idea that mind and body were separate entities, and this remained the accepted view of the human condition until as recently as the 1970s.

Medical practice is slow to change and, regrettably, there are still remnants of this reductionist mind versus body approach in our healthcare system – i.e. relying on what is known as the biomedical model, which focuses on purely biological factors and excludes psychological, environmental and social influences. However, we are now increasingly, as I say, moving towards a more nuanced, holistic approach – the bio-psycho-social model – and this is thanks in no small part to an enlightened American doctor and psychiatrist named George Engel.[2]

In 1977, Engel came up with the bio-psycho-social model after observing that doctors tended to see pain as a disease entity separate from man, something caused by an external factor. He also noted that patients themselves, regardless of their knowledge and education, tended to blame their illness on something that had happened *to* them, such as infection or a fall, and thought of pain as something almost apart from themselves.

The pain-as-separate-entity theory was an appealing one, at least for some practitioners, as it removed the necessity to deal with the emotional elements of a patient's problem. However, as Engel argued, pain is clearly something very much part of ourselves and it is impossible to treat it without looking at it in an integrated, 360-degree way.

SO WHAT IS THE BIO-PSYCHO-SOCIAL MODEL?

It is a medical approach that sees pain as an experience that results from the deep interrelation of three domains: biology, psychology and sociology.

That's it!

A simple sentence encapsulating a massive idea.

Biology (genetics, biochemistry), psychology (mood, personality, behaviour) and sociology (culture, family, socio-economics) are the three realms or domains that influence our physical and mental health. When the balance is lost between these three interlinking planes, pain and suffering occur. The ideal place to be is right at the intersection of the three circles – here is a pain-free world where you are able to cope with all of the internal and external factors in your life (see Figure 3 on p79). You juggle them like plates on sticks, managing them all without getting tired or stressed, or using up too much energy. Your universe is balanced. However, if you are not positioned happily in the centre of the three concentric circles – if one of the three elements is under strain or out of sync in some way – then you are likely to be suffering pain. The challenge for any physician is to work out from where in the system the pain is arising.

We are all unique and have vastly differing biological and genetic make-ups. This, together with the experiences we have and the influences exerted upon us throughout our lives, defines our ability to cope with our world. The degree to which we are sensitised or hardened by life depends on all of these elements and how they interact. And so, unsurprisingly, we all experience pain differently.

In the 1980s, John Loeser,[3] a neurosurgeon and pain researcher based in Washington, Seattle, devised his 'onion model' to demonstrate the individual's tolerance and experience of pain (see Figure 1 below). In it, the onion represents the pain experience and the layers that make up the onion put the pain in context. Interestingly, from his work in paediatrics, Loeser learned that even childhood experiences could modulate the pain experience into adulthood. Premature babies, for example, who routinely have to undergo more medical tests and painful procedures than those born at full term, have been found to be extra-sensitised to pain in adulthood (I go into more detail on this in Chapter 9). They also fear pain more. In addition, it has been well correlated that, due to their longer stays in hospital away from the love and physical contact of their parents, they associate pain with feelings of loss.

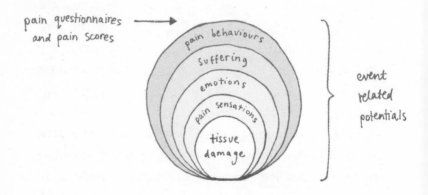

Figure 1: The 'onion model', demonstrating the individual's experience of pain

Pain exists deep inside us, and the practitioner, through history-taking and analysis, must work out which layer of the 'pain onion' they can peel away first to get to the cause: how are the elements of the pain overriding and controlling a return to normal? We may never be able to remove some elements but we can hopefully reduce their importance or simply eliminate the extra burden of minor ones so that the patient can cope once more.

PAIN AS A DISEASE OF THE NERVOUS SYSTEM

Remember earlier, when I said that pain occurs mostly on a neuro-psychological level? Well, what I meant by that was that pain exists predominantly in the nervous system and all its parts. In fact, it could be described as a disease of the nervous system.

Now, this may at first seem like a digression, but I am going to use an analogy here to explain how the nervous system works. It is essentially a sophisticated intelligence-gathering system, and to this extent it is very similar to the CIA. Both systems have a headquarters: for the CIA, it's Langley, and for the nervous system, it's the brain. The CIA's HQ is where all executive decisions are ultimately processed and made. And to make these decisions, HQ relies on a vast network of peripheral monitoring systems (satellite, video, audio, spy reports, encryption etc.) that feed into the centre from around the world, mainly through electronic channels. In the same way, nerves all over the body conduct their information to the brain by means of electrical impulses via the spinal cord which acts like a trunk cable channelling the messages to the brain.

Let's now look at where the intelligence gathering all starts, i.e. out there on the ground, where teams of field operatives, eavesdroppers and informers are constantly on the alert for intel about threats, potential or actual; in bodily terms, these guys are the sensors at the end of the nerves, and it is they who begin the collation of information and will report it to the station office if the amount of chatter is gathering momentum and could amount to 'a story'. It is then up to the station office to feed back any intel to the regional bureau (the spinal cord) where it will be evaluated for priority and validity. At this stage, a few senior staff may be woken up to assess the situation but, if it is decided that it is just a few unhappy locals kicking off rather than any real threat afoot, then everyone goes back to bed.

So, as you see, throughout this system there is a hierarchy of stops and checks through which the data goes before it is transmitted 'bottom up' for HQ's attention. All these reporting experts are employed for their innate ability as well as their experience and what they have learned along the way – any 'noise', disinformation and 'fake news' needs to be filtered out – and they will make snap decisions about what is important and what is not, accordingly.

Similarly, the nervous system will make a judgement about what to refer up to the brain, based on the context and quantity of information received, as well as its past experience. The entire nervous system behaves like a finely tuned, well-oiled intelligence agency that never sleeps, even when you do.

The medical word for all this, the body's incredible system for gathering intelligence about pain, is *nociception*, and it is crucial to the understanding of pain. As we will see, there is a big difference between nociception (which you could translate as 'the process of damaging-stimulus detection') and the actual conscious experience of pain. And yet this is an area of pain science that is poorly understood by many people, including most doctors, as very little time is spent on it in their training.

In order to survive the multiple threats to our existence, humans have evolved an extraordinary array of special senses and receptors to warn us of danger. These dangers may come in the form of chemical changes (internal or external), thermal changes (extreme temperatures, dry or humid climates), or mechanical changes (physical invasion, such as when our body is struck or pierced, perhaps by a stab wound or needle prick).

All of our special senses are backed up by vision, hearing, smell and taste, which can further inform the brain regarding the level and degree of threat. Moreover, our intricate memory system equips us with the ability not to repeat the action or event which harmed us. This manifests as fear, anxiety or avoidance.

Nociception is basically the neural process of taking the information provided by all these senses and receptors and encoding it to communicate and contribute information to the brain on the potential to cause pain. The information provided by nociception is not necessarily by itself enough to trigger the perception of pain. It is the brain which decides this ultimately, once it has processed the information.

To give an example: imagine you have just slammed your finger in a car door. If your reflex response is quick enough you will withdraw your arm, minimising damage to the tissues. However, the crush effect will be enough to initiate the release of inflammatory chemicals in the skin and tissues, irritating the very small nerves in them. The sensors in the nerves will detect this flood of chemicals and fire impulses up to the spinal cord.

At this point, the spinal cord will assess the level of noise coming from these nerves and initially do two things. Firstly, it will initiate the motor response of pulling your finger back from the source of the damage to prevent further injury. Secondly, it will conduct some of the information to the brain as a report of events, so that the brain can make an ongoing decision about how bad the injury is and what it needs to do to protect you. For example, does it need to send messages to the damaged tissue to cause it to swell, heal, or fight invading bugs? The brain will also make a fleeting assessment of the more long-term impact of the injury – how it will affect your ability to function and carry out daily activities, what threat it may pose to your long-term survival. These assessments are done by the brain's mood and emotional centres (the limbic centre) as well as the pre-frontal cortex. We know this because extensive research has been carried out, using fMRI technology, which has observed these parts of the brain 'light up' as pain is initiated. In some experiments, the effects of administering painful stimuli, such as hot lasers to the skin, in association with different emotions or pain-killing medicines, have been studied. And what these studies have shown is that the areas of the brain which light up change according to the stimulus.

If the healing mechanism for the crushed finger has been efficient and the tissues have recovered, the noise from the local nerves will settle, the spinal cord will lose interest and the brain will no longer be agitated. You won't notice the pain and can start using the finger again. All is well.

However, if the pain continues beyond a few hours the brain will become more agitated by it and continue with its evaluation. It will assess the injury in terms of how it will affect you and all aspects of your life – your job, caring for children or getting to work. *Will I have to take a day off, maybe a week? My boss will be furious, my team rely on me. I have a mortgage to pay, I can't afford this.* Depending on this assessment, the brain may cleverly depress your mood in order to slow you down as a protective measure. On the plains, back in the day, this sort of slow-down was important: it prevented or discouraged you from continuing to use an injured body part and gave you time to recover from a serious infection. Today, it is widely believed that, as part of our evolved socialisation and need for community, such depression or low mood is also a way of showing others in your social group that you are injured and in need of help. Additionally, it alerts you to the danger that lies in becoming isolated – today it translates as 'Why is Dad grumpy?'

But – and here's the amazing thing – even in the worst-case scenario, with the noise of nociception at full volume, and all our receptors firing like billy-o, the body has the ability to heal itself. And this is because we are capable of bioplasticity. In fact, we are bioplastic: the sensors in our receptors are constantly being replaced or modified. They have a short life of just a few days and, as new ones replace the old, so we can revert to our previous state. For example, through physiotherapy, the mechano-receptors (which are sensitive to movement) will change their sensitivity and type, as movement is restored and the brain allows the fear element to disperse.

What this means is that our current state of pain is not fixed. On the contrary: because we can have an effect on the replacement of those sensors and their sensitivity, *we can change our pain.*

For example, if you twist your ankle and tear a ligament in it, yes, it will swell and immediately hurt. The sensors in the ligament and surrounding tissues will start firing all sorts of messages to the spinal cord about the state of the tissue and how badly it is injured. Chemicals released by the injured cells will leak onto sensitive nerves, which will send signals, and pain will be felt. It may be intense enough that you will hobble and stop using the joint to prevent further injury. In return, and at the same time, the brain will mobilise all of the inflammatory and healing chemicals and cells necessary to activate healing. This will continue for three weeks or so, during which time the swelling will subside as it is no longer needed, and, as the cells heal, the production of pain-sensitising chemicals will decrease. The receptors needed for the alarm state will no longer be necessary, and the brain will stop responding.

As you begin to use the ankle again, there will be a transition stage at the receptor level. When loaded with weight, the ankle will feel stiff as the stretch receptors wake up and more receptors are made by the cells to monitor and regulate movement. Once the brain has assessed that the load and movement are not dangerous and causing more injury, it will allow you to be more active. The local mechano-receptors will change from being ones of alarm to ones of movement and activity.

○ ○ ○

You may have noticed that I have omitted to mention one particular type of receptor – pain receptors. That is because we don't have any! Nor do we have any 'pain nerves' or 'pain pathways' or 'pain centres'.

And that is because, as I suggested earlier, pain is what we experience once the brain has decided to notice it – usually as a result of it realising that the stimulus is actually or potentially dangerous and when it wants us to realise that some sort of protective response is necessary. And the brain's decision to notice pain is brought about not just by sensors in our tissues but by the messages from them being filtered and added to by other parts of the nervous system, which assess, modify and decide on whether to make it a problem for us. Our bodies have a network of stations feeding into a 'decision' regarding whether to 'hurt'.

Effectively, *only* the brain can truly experience hurt or suffering. You might have to think about that one for a minute.

And yet, even more strangely, if I made a neat slice through your cranium right now, flipped your skull open and stabbed you in the brain with a pencil, you wouldn't feel any pain at all. Any pain you did feel would not be coming from the brain tissue itself but from the damaged nociceptive receptors in the skin, membranes and bone surfaces of the skull that surround it. Brain tissue contains no nociceptive receptors at all. Indeed, we make use of this fact every day in brain surgery, when patients are often awake during an operation, to help the surgeon avoid important territories which would be catastrophic if cut. This is why it may be surprising to hear that brain tumours very rarely present with headache as their main symptom. It is only when the tumour compresses important structures, preventing them from functioning properly, that the first symptoms, such as mood change or epilepsy, tend to occur.

There are two posited explanations for the lack of pain sensation in the brain. Firstly, the brain and spinal cord develop separately from the peripheral nerves of the body at embryo stage and so none of the three main types of nociceptor (mechanical, thermal and chemical) exist in the brain. Anthropologists believe that nature probably also decided that, by the time such receptors were being fired, it was 'Goodnight Vienna' anyway, as the degree of damage to 'mission control' was too great and so the space taken up by these receptors was better used for other functions.

But then why do we get headaches? Because there are plenty of pain-sensitive structures in the head and neck which can refer pain around the eyes and skull. Headaches are not actually of brain origin.

As I say, pain is what we experience once the brain has decided to notice it. And so it is that most of the time the body's sensory and nervous systems will respond to 'damage' stimuli without us ever actually knowing it. It is only when the brain deems it necessary to 'express' these messages and when their summation is enough, that it will bring the problem to our attention consciously, either as a physical reaction (withdraw finger from flame) or as the experience of pain.

In summary, all of these systems are ultimately designed to alert us, raise the alarm in us or, most importantly, protect us. So, though it may be hard to believe, pain is actually good. We know this thanks to a very small group of special but unfortunate individuals who cannot feel pain at all. Some of them don't live very long and most are besieged by problems they cannot detect as they do not have internal alarm systems (of this, more later.) On a philosophical level, one can also say that pain is important simply because it confirms we exist. Pain and suffering are part of the human condition.

○ ○ ○

Why is it, then, that some people seem to feel pain more intensely than others? René Descartes believed that pain intensity and type were correlated quite simply with the degree and extent of tissue damage. For example, the more a needle is pressed into the skin the more the pain perceived, regardless of who the individual is experiencing the pain. However, this theory was disproved by research carried out in 1956 by Dr Henry K. Beecher,[4] a pioneering military anaesthetist. He compared a number of severely wounded soldiers with a civilian group, and found that less than a quarter of the soldiers had requested any pain relief in the form of morphine, compared to 83 per cent of the civilian group. The troops may of course have just been 'tougher', and there was a possibility, according to Beecher, that the soldiers' ability to cope was also due to the context of the pain, in that for many of them their wound meant that they were out of the fight, they were going home and at least they weren't dead! But this could not possibly account entirely for how little pain relief the soldiers seemed to need. The study showed that there is actually little correlation between the extent of a pathological wound and the pain experienced.

In 1965, neurobiologist Patrick Wall and psychologist Ronald Melzack got much closer to a viable concept of how pain is perceived and controlled by the central nervous system and spinal cord.[5] Their idea came to be known as the 'gate theory of pain'. It worked on the premise that groups of nerve cells opened and closed 'gates', thereby determining whether messages could pass through or not. This also allowed for the idea that there had to be sufficient messages to reach a 'threshold' before the central nervous system recognised them. And it showed that there were other processes and factors that determined how and when pain was felt.

In addition, Wall and Melzack experimented with using different stimuli to confuse the brain. They played around with setting contexts around pain stimulation, for example using stress and fear to see if there was a change in the level of pain the subjects reported, which there was. This research provided some insight into the curious fact that pain can continue long after the initial injury has healed, or even exist without injury or a disease process in the first place – a conundrum which has been wonderfully expressed by Dr Fabrizio Benedetti, professor of physiology and neuroscience at the University of Turin,[6] and an expert on placebos, who succinctly states: 'Pain is the product of bottom-up processes and top-down modulation.'

In this chapter we have covered the 'bottom-up' process of pain — i.e. nociception, the nervous system's sensory response to harmful stimuli – and in the next we will look at the 'top-down' bit, that is, how the brain experiences pain, how it reacts, as well as how it is that we can be in pain but not have any discernible physical cause or reason for it.

CHAPTER 2

WHEN PAIN BECOMES A HABIT

'Realise that everything connects to everything else.'
– Leonardo da Vinci

You will remember in the last chapter we saw that pain is what we experience once the brain has decided that an injury or any other source of pain is sufficiently serious to be causing us a problem. But why, then, does the brain sometimes continue to register pain even when an injury has long since healed?

Many people (currently some 43 per cent of the UK adult population) experience pain that goes on for longer than three months and which may continue for years despite there being no structural or organic injury to which it can be attributed.[7] These are the patients who have normal X-rays, MRIs and blood tests but who still feel debilitating pain. How can this be?

Let's go back to HQ. Its role is to take all of the information deemed to be important at station office and bureau level and respond to it. In the first instance, this may be to monitor the aftermath of a local riot (finger injury or wound) and decide whether it is all settling nicely or if it represents a gathering political trend or activist group who are going to cause trouble (maybe an infection in the wound).

HQ also uses experience of past events to understand the context around the riot (injury). What happened in the past can augur the degree of alarm felt. And HQ may need to bring in other departments to assess the meaning and risk from the riot. In physical terms, this would commonly be the emotional and cognitive centres, those able to think through what it all means: i.e. how important is the injury likely to be? For example, if you are a guitar player or surgeon, a finger injury is potentially more of a disaster than if you are a singer or an optician.

As we have discussed, usually the nociception noise settles as the injury heals, and the HQ alarm status subsides. At most, a memory of the injury or the action which led to it will be stored or logged for future quick response. It will be tagged. So, too, the key departments necessary to deal with it will be remembered for quick mobilisation. The whole event will leave a response 'signature' that is unique to each event. In pain science we call this a 'neuro-signature' (remember this word: we will come back to it shortly).

Most injuries to a healthy body, including bone fractures, will heal in four to six weeks, and we would not expect the nociception associated with them to continue much longer than that. Sometimes inflammation and the nerves around the injury can continue to cause pain for a while, but it is generally accepted that *all healing* will

ve taken place within three months. This is considered
o be the point past which, if pain is still felt, it assumes the
definition of 'chronic' (in the sense of lasting longer than
expected, rather than very bad).

What we now know is that, if pain persists for long
enough and other fear associations, contexts or memories
get attached to it through a filter of sensitisers such as age,
gender and previous trauma, as well as childhood and prior
experiences, then it can get established rather like a bad
habit. Scientists refer to this sort of negative peripheral
experience around pain as a raised 'signal to noise ratio',
which results in increased activation of calcium channels
in the nervous system, which in turn boosts the number of
messages travelling around and between nerve cells. This
is thought to be responsible for 'central sensitisation', a
phenomenon first described by a brilliant anaesthetist and
neurobiologist, Dr Clifford Woolf, at University College
London, in 1983.[8] Central sensitisation is defined as an
'amplification of neural signalling in the central nervous
system that elicits pain hypersensitivity', and is the process
by which the brain becomes involved in prolonged stimulation from inflammation in the tissues in the periphery. Basically, it turns up the volume and intensity on
everything. An American study carried out more recently,
in 2009, showed that in people who had neck pain from
injured muscles, other parts of their body (legs and arms)
also became more sensitive to touch, and that when the
neck muscles were injected with painkillers, the other parts
became less tender to the touch too.[9]

Woolf argued that central sensitisation has three effects:
it lowers the firing threshold of the nerves; it causes the

after-effects of pain to linger; and it causes incoming impulses from surrounding tissues to be seen as noxious even when they are not. It is effectively a type of neurobiological 'learning disorder' in which the brain misinterpretes and logs messages and cannot change direction. Some scientists liken it to a form of classical conditioning. Just as Pavlov's dogs learned to salivate in response to a bell, so the nervous system becomes sensitised to respond to small stimuli with chronic pain.

Neurones in the brain can form the synapses (junctions) for these habit pathways extremely quickly. Research has shown that a neurone can actually move up to 30 per cent of its length, by an amoeboid type action of twisting and writhing towards another neurone with which it wants to link. The direction it has to face is dictated by a chemical messenger, emitted by the other neurone inviting it to hook up. Each neurone can also form as many sprouts from its body to link up with as many other neurones as it wants to. This works on an exponential basis, spreading out in all directions, and so a multitude of possibilities for connections is possible, enabling the brain to learn, adapt and change very fast. As Professor V Ramachandran, a neurobiologist at UCL, explained in a recent TED talk,[10] 'The brain contains 100 billion neurones, each one of which can make 1000–10,000 connections. This exceeds the number of elementary particles in the universe.' Indeed, babies can form 3 million new synapses every second, all of which would fit on the end of a pin.

These billions of interconnecting neurones sit in a soup of immune and vascular cells which communicate with each other through intricate electrochemical and molecular mechanisms. Some cells connect, some supply and support and some protect. The brain constantly terminates, rebuilds and enhances these connections through a lifelong process of remodification, which is necessary for us to survive as our environment changes and places different demands on us. The connections compete with each other for survival. Some die off as they are no longer needed, and new, more relevant ones are formed.

The trouble is that, while these networks can be formed pretty quickly, they may not break so readily, and the longer they experience pain, the more likely this will lead to changes in the brain's structure, the most serious of which is atrophy (shrinkage) of the 'grey matter'. This discovery was made by Professor Vania Apkarian in a study at Northwestern University's Feinberg School of Medicine into the source of pain and its cognitive effect.[11] Grey matter, so named because it does actually have a greyish hue, comprises the regions of the brain involved in muscle control and sensory perception, such as seeing and hearing, memory, emotions, speech, decision-making and self-control. And shrinkage of grey matter will cause patients with chronic pain who are also stressed or depressed to exhibit a 'withdrawal' pattern of behaviour, to become guarded and socially isolated and have trouble sleeping. Social withdrawal, too, can become a vicious cycle because the more it develops in the patient, the more they feel pain and in turn become increasingly withdrawn. Depression and pain are intimately intertwined in a dance of causation.

In their research, Apkarian and his team showed that, with extended exposure to chronic pain, instead of just responding to a period of externally generated impulses and then returning to a more resting state, the brain would begin to take on the pain itself. Furthermore, if the chronic pain lasted more than five years, the brain would lose between 5 and 11 per cent of grey matter density. This was particularly true of a part of the brain called the hippocampus, which is responsible for forming and associating memories. In those subjects who had had years of pain, the hippocampus was distinctly smaller. The pain also seemed to have set up a new and unusual link between two other parts of the brain: the pre-frontal cortex (which processes sensory information such as what hurts, how much and what it means) and the nucleus accumbens (which processes motivation and pleasure). The outcome of these two regions talking to each other was a diminution of the person's ability to make decisions and function properly. Further research is needed to show whether blocking the development or transmission of signals between these two regions can help to prevent chronic pain developing.

It might be helpful here to think of the brain as essentially a linked network of regions – a bit like the London tube map. The stations are the many brain centres (known as 'ignition nodes'), connected by the tube lines, i.e. the neuronal pathways. Imagine using different coloured pens to highlight the various routes from your friends' houses to yours. Each friend has a unique route passing through different stations and changing at different stops. Using the term coined by Professor Patrick Wall, we call each of these routes or pathways a pain 'neurosignature'. Each neurosignature is an etched 'memory' of a pain, which may be new or old, active or dormant, and it is logged in the substance or matrix of the brain. If the route is used regularly then it will remain active. If not, it will begin to fade – just as the memory of a tube route might fade if you did not make the journey so frequently.

However, if at any stage one of the nodes along a route is stimulated, it can trigger all of the route or neurosignature to fire up, thereby sparking the experience of that unique pain. As an example, let's say you fractured a wrist bone years ago when you were knocked over by a mugger. He gets away with your bag, containing your wallet with money and a sentimental photograph of a loved one in it. He also gets your phone. So now you are sitting there, on a cold wet pavement, somewhat shocked, cradling your wrist. It's dark and you are some way from home. The street is quiet and you are worried that the assailant might come back or someone else might take advantage of you. You have the embarrassment of knocking on someone's door to ask for help. The wrist is beginning to throb and ache and every movement hurts. Nociception fires up with a vengeance, sending negative injury messages to your nervous system and brain, and your brain accepts that pain is appropriate.

Let's suppose you get help, that you get to A&E and they cast your wrist and that, six weeks later, the wrist is healed and the pain has all but gone. It's been a massive inconvenience at work, and replacing your keys, wallet and cards has been a hassle. But you're OK. Except that, despite the healing, your brain has etched and logged a neurosignature around the whole event, linking several key ignition nodes. The route or signature between these centres is now highlighted without you even being conscious of it. Fast-forward two years and most of the time your wrist remains pain-free. However, you notice that whenever it is winter and dark, cold and wet, you get a deep ache in the wrist. The familiar smell of wet leaves reminds you of that night. Your route home has not changed so you always get that little jolt of memory of when and where you were jumped, and you still look over your shoulder. Carrying your bag seems to make the ache come back. We can see that the key ignition nodes here are the smell, vision and hearing memory centres: the hippocampus which links the memory with the place and time, and the amygdala and limbic centres which re-invoke the twang of fear – 'what if' – and of indignation – 'why me?' Meanwhile, the pre-frontal cortex is busy making decisions about what to do if another mugger jumps out and the sympathetic nervous system still seems to raise your pulse and breathing rate, preparing you for flight or fight. These are all part of a single event, but each node, if stimulated, can fire the whole experience, and pain in your wrist is the result, even though the injury is long healed and nociception is long over.

And so, rather like smoking, pain can effectively become a habit that the brain gets into and which it cannot break. It becomes a 'closed loop' or 'default mode' of repetitive pathways which is difficult to re-route.

In his excellent book *The Power of Habit*, Charles Duhigg cites research in which the habit of smoking can be visualised in patients' brains via fMRI imaging.[12] The pathway of the 'smoking-habit' brain centres literally light up. If these same patients are scanned later, after they have quit smoking, there is a new and alternative 'smoking-free' pathway which is also lit up, but the 'habit signature' is still there. The fact that an old habit pathway still exists explains why it is so easy to fall back into that habit if, for some reason, it is re-ignited – for example, by a stress trigger.

Pain behaves in the same way. Even after the patient has conquered their pain, its old signature is still there to be awakened if a particular node on that network is triggered. The neurosignature is believed to be a protective mechanism given to us by nature so that we have the memory of an experience should we be re-exposed to any element of it in the future. It is predominantly there to recognise danger.

We now know that almost all responses in the brain rely on multiple linked areas that are processed together, not just isolated specialist regions. This infinite network is known in neuroscience as the 'connectome'. It is the connections that are the key, much as they are between humans: when we become isolated, we cease to function. As Stevie Wonder once said: 'You need the team to make the dream.'

○ ○ ○

To recap, nociception is going on as a process all the time in us as an assessment of our environment, but we don't feel it as pain unless one of our senses is so stimulated and reaches such a high threshold that it requires action from the brain to protect itself – for example, withdrawing a finger from a flame. These thresholds are different in all of us, as is the length of time we can tolerate them.

To nail the concept of neurosignature once and for all, let's go back one more time to HQ.

Let's suppose that instead of a few locals kicking off, or a roadside bomb exploding in a distant land, the big one hits. For some months the local offices have been sending reports of multiple intel about an impending strike. They have heard it's going to be big; the only problem is they don't know where it's going to occur. Then – boom! – someone plants a device right in the heart of Langley. Safe, highly fortified HQ goes down. Half the building is gone and dozens are killed. Systems fail. Communications are lost. Panic, disbelief. Every system and department is mobilised to seal the breach, contain the damage and assess further threat.

With time, of course, the walls are rebuilt, the glass replaced, staff positions filled and systems restored. But is HQ ever really the same again? Everyone remembers and mourns. New regimes are put in place – no complacency now – and the atmosphere changes. The local offices become twitchier to spies and regional movements and file reports more frequently. At the same time, HQ demands more intel and overreacts to small events. Danger is everywhere.

This heightened security situation equates, in bodily terms, to a serious injury – a brain or spinal injury or multiple injuries sustained in a serious traffic accident. After the initial injuries heal, the scars fade, but the victim is never quite the same again. The old wound aches, particularly in wet weather, one's fatigue won't improve, movements hurt. Sleep is disturbed, mood is low, libido wanes. Passing the scene of the accident raises the pulse and a cold sweat descends. The victim avoids crowds and not going out seems easier. The dog gets kicked, a partner gets snapped at. Work has been patient but it all seems too hard. The pain becomes a reason to withdraw. The neurosignature is set.

The peripheral nerves (bottom-up), though healed, will still fire messages of concern because they have been sensitised to be on alert, not just by all the nociception, but from the neurosignature: now, any small movement or sensory information (heat, touch) can set off inappropriate levels of pain. And the more the nerves fire, the more pain is felt, which in turn further sensitises them.

For a long time, it was thought that nerves were one-way systems like electrical wires, but we now know that they are capable of two-way chatter. The receptors fire information to the spinal cord, which reacts by sending more messages back down into the tissues. There is a two-way chat between them. In this way, the pain can become a vicious cycle or habit at a local level. Furthermore, the nerves connect by synapses with other types of nerves, which feed information into the loop. As a result, the chatter spreads throughout the system, further sensitising it. For example, in addition to local inflammation in the injured tissues, such as swelling and redness, the nerves can send a response around the body. This is why people with a trapped nerve in their low back can get a swollen foot as well as a debilitating pain in the leg. We call this *peripheral sensitisation*. The nerve is compressed in the low back by a disc protruding onto it and interfering with its conduction. As a result, the two-way chatter to the spinal cord is impaired and an alarm state is induced to promote action from the brain. But the brain is not aware of where exactly the nerve is irritated, it just knows that the region that this nerve supplies is the foot, and the foot is sending it alarm signals. At the same time, the nerve itself becomes irritated by impaired cell function and elicits an inflammatory response in the area of the body supplied by it – in this case the foot. Consequently, the foot can swell and redden even though no healing response is actually needed.

○ ○ ○

So, as you can see, once the pain signature has become established, and has been influenced by all our life experiences, as far back as our childhood, as well as all our perceived conceptions of the world, real or not, pain can become ingrained and cyclical, and move around the body. A good example of this kind of central nervous system sensitisation is irritable bowel syndrome (IBS). People with this condition not only suffer unpleasant symptoms such as changes in their bowel habits, pain and bloating, but are also more likely to experience pain in other parts of their body, such as fibromyalgia (characterised by global muscle pain), chronic fatigue or migraines (see Chapter 7 for more on these).

It is quite clear that, throughout our lives, many other factors in our environment sensitise us and lower our pain threshold. And research has shown that these factors potentiate pain outside of anything structural or genetic. As we will see in Chapter 4 – How Stress Makes us Hurt – nature does not provide a blueprint that defines our whole being but rather an intricate 'super-system' that we engage to respond to the stresses of the environment in which we live. This comprises the psyche, as well as endocrine (glandular), neurological and immune systems, and is mediated predominantly through chemical messages transmitted between our cells. When our super-system ceases to function properly, the result is pain, illness and disease.

Pain is in a sense a mode of perception used by the body to tell us that something is wrong. As Dr Gabor Maté puts it:[13]

> Physiologically the pain pathways channel information that we have blocked from reaching us by more direct routes. Pain is a powerful secondary mode of perception to alert us when our primary modes have shut down. It provides us with data that we ignore at our peril.

Getting to the heart of what this 'data' of pain really means and understanding the messages it is trying to give us is what the following chapters are about. I hope that you will find it an interesting and enlightening journey.

CASE HISTORY: MAGGIE

Throughout this book, I am going to illustrate the points I am explaining with the stories of real patients. I will tell you a bit about their background, and why they came to my clinic, and I will try to show you how almost all of them got better by understanding and overcoming their pain. Naturally, I have changed names and identifying details to preserve patient confidentiality, but the examples I give are all real.

Let's start with Maggie, a patient of mine who was 65 when I first saw her in my clinic. Maggie is an intelligent woman who worked in high-level administration in a large hospital before she retired. She has lived alone since she was widowed.

She came to see me after she had slipped in the winter snow six months previously and broken her left knee. The break was across the joint, where the lower leg bone takes all the load of the knee. The fracture was not displaced, so the hospital decided to let it heal without surgery. But Maggie had been splinted for too long due to miscommunication between the medical experts treating her. And she was now experiencing a lot of pain and needed to use a crutch. She felt that the pain was travelling up her left side into her back and neck like 'creeping rot'. She had not been offered sufficient physiotherapy before she was discharged.

By the time she came to see me, she was scared to go out and saw only a bleak future of pain and loneliness ahead. An old tendency to the 'black dog' of depression had begun to take hold. Up until her accident, she had loved travelling – she'd just been on holiday to New Zealand – and she had been fearless of all that the world could throw at her. But now that had all been taken away, and to top it all, she was seeing less of her usual companions as they continued to enjoy their lives.

Since the initial fracture she had become much less active and lost muscle bulk and tone as well as the ability to keep her balance, which is particularly significant in people aged over 65. In her very much weakened state, the likely progression for her would be to go on to have another fall and possibly break a hip or worse. Once bedridden, she would be more likely to get a chest or kidney infection, which could prove fatal. I feared the chronic pain Maggie was experiencing could literally be the death of her unless we could turn her around both physically and psychologically.

The answer lay in working with all the elements of Maggie's pain – the biological, the social and the psychological. My first task was to convince her that we were there for her and to contact us if there were any crises. She worried constantly about falling while getting to the shops. She missed her husband terribly. We discussed him and how he would have wanted her to forge on. We also agreed the not unreasonable target of going on holiday in a year's time, as it was her passion. Just embracing this slightly lifted her mood. I explained that despite what she felt – the pain expanding and becoming much worse – the initial injury, painful and poorly treated as it was, had, in fact, healed in the intervening six months. That's what bone and tissue does without any help. This reassurance along with some gentle mobilisation of her leg gave her the confidence to put more weight on it almost instantly.

What she was now dealing with were the top-down processes of the neurosignature formed in her brain around the injury and resultant continuing pain. The 'nodes' of the pain experience were multiple. Firstly, psychological in the form of anger at having been given poor treatment and being left to manage; fear at what the future held and being unable to move without pain; a feeling of loss of her friends, who seemed not to care, and of her husband, who would have looked after her, taken control and known what to do. She resented her swollen knee and saw it as a disfigurement on her body. She refused to move it, because it was broken and distorted in her eyes. Secondly, there was the social element: she was estranged from her brother, she was too proud to ask for help and her friends had stopped calling. She lived in a high-rise flat where the lift did not always work. Her landlord had been unsupportive. And thirdly, the biological one: she still had some swelling in the knee due to inactivity and poor drainage. The tissues were tight and sore and the muscles had wasted. Any one of those factors would re-ignite her pain if she thought about them.

There was a change in Maggie and her leg pain from the very first appointment. Manual examination and mobilisation had already enabled some new, pain-free movement. It had also rid her of her back pain, which had developed as she compensated for her painful gait. She would need a few more sessions to accelerate her mobility. But Maggie now knew what her goals were and the strategy she had to follow to achieve them. She was armed with a range of exercises, paced and staged, and the right pain relief to enable her to get going and stop fearing movement. She was to set up a gym membership because she would eventually need weights to strengthen her muscles. Most importantly, she had a clearer view of what was going on, having had explained to her what was causing her pain and that it did not mean 'harm'.

I am happy to report that Maggie reached out to her friends, who were very saddened to hear that she had been suffering in silence, and she has just booked a trip to Chile with them.

CHAPTER 3

WELCOME TO LIFE ON PLANET STRESS

'The human organism is the most complex and
extraordinary entity in the known Universe.'
– Hans Selye, *The Stress of Life*

Picture, if you will, the opening scene from *Bambi*. A
young inexperienced deer is grazing the forest floor under a
green canopy of trees. His head is down, rooting for acorns
and seeds. Subconsciously, though, his nose is constantly
sampling the air, while his ears, like mobile antennae, scan
for suspicious or threatening noises. His brain has adapted
to the subtle ambient tunes of the wood and pushed them
to the background of awareness, as they are deemed not to
be a threat. While his eyes are on the floor, he cannot use
them to spot predators, so his ears are everything. They
can determine where a sound is coming from, and how far
away it is, and will triangulate the threat even when it is
obscured by a bush or tree.

Suddenly the tranquility is broken by the snap of a twig.
He freezes even before he can respond. He uses his ears to

locate the noise and focuses his eyes to assess the danger. He breathes slowly through his nose, scenting the air. His pulse quickens and his muscles tense, readying him for action. His forebrain shuts down; there's no time for thinking about anything except which way to run. Thinking could be fatal. After a moment of intense alertness during which he senses no attack is imminent, he stands down and returns to grazing, but now raising his head up more frequently to survey the landscape. He is twitchier now. He is sensitised.

His brain makes the natural percentage decision that the longer there is no attack, the less likely it is. This time there is no threat.

But now imagine the same scene, this time with a wolf breaking cover, ears back, teeth snarling. Bambi's freeze turns into a desperate run in the opposite direction. He cuts himself and strikes objects, even breaks a toe, but nothing slows him; he feels no pain – why? Because whatever injury he has is infinitely less serious than being dead; pain at this moment would be an unnecessary distraction from mortal danger. Eventually he outruns the wolf, who skulks off, disappointed. To Bambi's small and primitive brain, it is a crisis response soon over, a percentage game: survive or die. His wounds heal, and compared to being dead the pain is a trifle. He will continue to graze and think deer-like thoughts because he will not be worried or distracted by what *might* happen; just by what he knows to be happening now and its level of imminent danger to his survival.

○ ○ ○

These two scenarios illustrate how pain is mediated by context and the level of stress.

When Bambi breaks a toe or even a leg while fleeing from death, he keeps going, unaware of his injury. Unless the limb has completely buckled and he is unable to support his weight, he will carry on running until he has either escaped or been caught. This phenomenon is called stress-induced analgesia. The brain mobilises its own internal pain relief system based on naturally made opiate chemicals. These chemicals flood all of the relevant synapses involved in the response, blocking the pain. There have been many instances of athletes and soldiers who have suffered serious injuries but have only become conscious of them once they have completed their event or task. For example, soldiers who have had a leg blown off by a land mine have been known to try to get up and walk, unaware of the gravity of their injuries. This is why the first thing an army field medic does when attending an injured soldier is to explain what has happened.

When I was thrown across the bonnet of a car while riding my moped in London recently, the first thing the ambulance crew said to me when they arrived on the scene was: 'You've been in a road accident.' Stating the obvious, you might think – but necessary. At that point, due to stress-induced analgesia, I was feeling no pain from my injuries and, as we saw with Bambi, my forebrain and emotional centres had shut down while my body dealt with the level of threat to my life.

A contrasting response kicks in once the chase is over. Satisfied that the impending danger has gone, the brain allows the incoming flood of nociception to make its presence felt and starts to assess the effects on the body. Now follows a period of stress-induced *hyperalgesia*, when the level of pain becomes all-consuming and is escalated by the realisation that the injury is serious and in its own way threatening. Fear and meaning become involved.

A few hours after my moped accident, my body began to ache and bruises started to appear as my brain allowed a flood of messages from all the tissue receptors in my muscles to establish themselves as pain. Thankfully, I had no serious injuries, but even if I had, I would have been protected from the knowledge of this until then – i.e. after the crisis had passed. It was only at this point that my forebrain and all of the other emotional centres I had switched off kicked in, catastrophising about what might have happened and the possible impact on my work and my family.

○ ○ ○

To understand why we humans need a stress response and how it makes us behave the way we do, we need to go back to prehistoric times, when our ancestors regularly came face to face with fearsome creatures that made them, like Bambi, freeze or flee. Over time we learned how to use our guile to survive each day; we found safety, protection and power in social groups with whom we could hunt, feed and mate. We even thrived on episodes of high adrenaline, as these kept us alert, sharp, lean and quick. And as Neanderthals gave way to *Homo sapiens* some 70,000 years ago, we developed altruistic behaviour, such as grooming and nursing, to prevent disease and aid recovery. We learned that if we let the best fighter or hunter die, we endangered the whole tribe because it prevented his knowledge from being passed on to others and from protecting us in the future. So, the tribe took care of him. Anthropologists have found in many *sapiens* skeletons evidence of major long bone fractures that have clearly healed. This shows that the victim was not left as a sacrificial meal for a lion; he was nursed back to health by the tribe.

Propagation of the gene through survival and sex produced the two key drivers to our existence: fear and lust. Arguably they drive us still, only tempered and tamed by the overlay of modern societal rules. However, we must remember that the environment in which we now live is very different from the one from which we evolved. We evolved over millions of years, but the changes in our more recent history – the development of agriculture 12,000 years ago, and the industrial revolution only 200 years ago – have occurred in such a relatively short time that we have not yet been able to fully adapt to them. As a result, much of our bio-psychology is poorly suited to our current environment.

In the modern, developed Western world, we no longer daily face the sort of mortal dangers that we did in the past, and yet we remain as competitive as we always were. According to Professor Jean Twenge, head of psychology at San Diego University, we are now physically the safest we have ever been but our children are the most emotionally fragile they have ever been.[14] Think about that for a moment – because it bodes badly for our experience of pain, among other things, in the future.

The stress response is fundamentally a mechanism we

developed to adapt to our environment, to improve our chances of survival. The stressors then were mostly physical, involving running from attack, fighting, competing, gathering and, latterly, farming. They often represented real mortal threat and danger. By comparison, other worries based on social competition and jostling for position in the hierarchy were mere niggles.

And yet now, worries to do with social competition and the like are among our main stressors. These days we have very little in our environment to adapt and respond to, except on a cognitive and intellectual level. We have lost context in relation to fearful events and now, it could be argued, we fear almost anything we simply don't like. We have become over-sensitised to trivial – even subliminal – worries.

What's more, as primitive brains grew and developed with each successive generation, humans not only developed an awareness of danger but, crucially, how to anticipate it – a uniquely human trait. And from this anticipation came anxiety, the fear of what *might* happen. Their offspring started to be born 'pre-loaded' with certain neuropsychological software designed to protect them, and hardwired to respond in certain ways. These traits are known in neuropsychology as 'biases' and they strongly affect the way we live our lives.

One important example is what we now call negativity bias – this is where we attach more importance to the seriousness of something happening than to the likelihood of it occurring. Back in prehistory, it saved our lives, but in modern times it flaws our decision-making and affects our ability to take risks.

Let's imagine that one day, back in the time of early man, you went to the watering hole and found a sabre-toothed tiger there. Would you decide never to go back, to avoid the risk of being eaten, or would you risk it because you needed a drink? The effect of negativity bias in our decision-making would dictate that we would rather die of thirst by slow dehydration than risk a painful but quick death at the hands of a predator. The horror of being eaten outweighs the less certain and less painful death by parching. Contemporary research into decision-making by humans today has confirmed this bias: anthropological analysis of hominid remains has been done which shows dehydration of tissues before death.

Anthropologists have discerned that early man could make one of two mistakes in this situation: he could think either that a tiger was lurking in the bushes when it actually was not, or that there was no tiger in the bushes when there actually was. The cost of the first was a life of needless anxiety while the cost of the second was death. Needless to say, we are descended from the ones in the first group – the anxiety-prone ones, who avoided death long enough to procreate. The bolder strain of early man who ran the risk of being eaten by the tiger probably didn't live long enough to pass on his genes. As a result, the default setting of the modern brain is to overestimate threats and underestimate opportunities, and also underestimate our resources to cope with threat and to fulfil those opportunities.

Unfortunately, this anxiety-prone behaviour then gets amplified by another hard-wired setting, confirmation bias, which is the tendency to search for, interpret, favour or recall information in a way that confirms our pre-existing beliefs or ideas. The more we worry about something, the more we believe it to be true. Thus we become preoccupied with threats which at first seemed small and manageable. I will come back to this later, when I talk about what stresses us in modern life.

So do we even need this stress response any more? Yes, because if you need to be alert to a threat or danger, like any normal mammal dealing with an acute emergency, and you cannot activate the stress response, you are in big trouble. In people with conditions such as Addison's disease and Shy-Drager syndrome, who are unable to secrete vital stress hormones, this becomes all too apparent. When confronted with an acute stress like a car accident, they cannot maintain their blood pressure and go into shock.

But equally damaging, and much more common, is an excess of stress hormones. When we are sitting in traffic, endlessly worrying about mortgage payments or fretting about a bullying boss, and are unable to switch off the stress response, we risk serious damage to our health.

And this is where stress and pain meet. Stress is fundamentally linked to pain and illness and, if not addressed, can go on to cause disease. Like pain, it arises when we can no longer cope with an imbalance that has developed between ourselves and the three elements or domains of our environment (see Figure 3 at the end of this chapter): society, biology and psychology. And I feel passionately that a deeper understanding of the mechanisms of stress can not only benefit professionals – doctors, coaches, policy makers – who in turn will be able to treat illness effectively, but also provide a new philosophy to guide us all within the laws of nature and help us improve the way we live.

Like most mammals, we humans are generally able to maintain our internal environment very successfully – i.e. the composition of our body chemistry remains remarkably constant – despite all the changes around us. For example, even when exposed to extremes of heat or cold, our body temperature does not vary. And the way it does this is by a process called homeostasis. This is what ensures that our internal environment is maintained and regulated against whatever our external one throws at us.

A stressor is anything in the outside environment which knocks us out of homeostatic balance. And the stress response is what our body does to re-establish this balance. For most animals, the stress mechanism is not only what maintains their health but helps them stay alive. Their bodies' physiological responses are superbly adapted to dealing with short-term physical emergencies, for example being chased by a predator. For the vast majority of beasts, stress is about a short-term crisis which ends in either survival or death.

But for *Homo sapiens* it's different. As we evolved and adapted, our new-found cerebral and emotional abilities brought with them more angst, and more to process. Our ability to cope began to be tested in new ways as we had to mobilise many more subtle physiological responses to manage an ongoing, unrelenting type of stress – and ultimately our coping mechanism began to be eroded if it was tested for too long. To reflect this, Bruce McEwen, a neuroscientist at Rockefeller University, expanded the idea of homeostasis into allostasis, whereby rather than our having specific responses to specific stressors, stress actually has a more wide-reaching effect on us, with myriad adjustments being made throughout different systems in the body to address the shift in balance.[15] He coined the term 'allostatic load' to describe the micro wear-and-tear which ensues as a result of a continued assault on our internal control mechanisms and to explain how, if this becomes damaging enough, the system will fail.

As Professor Robert Sapolsky, a researcher and author on stress at Stanford University says: 'This is the essence of what stress does. No single disastrous effect, no lone gunman. Instead, kicking, poking, impeding here and there, make this a bit worse, that a bit less effective. Thus, making it a bit more likely for the roof to cave in at some point.' [16]

This combined and global effect of stress has been demonstrated in numerous studies, including one carried out by military researchers many years ago which looked at the cardiac health of soldiers who had seen intense active combat.[17] One cohort of subjects comprised veterans from the Second World War and the other veterans from the Vietnam War, some of whom were just 19 years old. Comparing the two cohorts, the researchers found that the physiological condition of the hearts of the soldiers who had fought in Vietnam was poorer for their age than those of the Second World War soldiers – indeed, the Vietnam veterans' hearts were like those of 50-year-olds who had not seen combat in a normal population.

The researchers worked out that, although the WW2 veterans had seen intense and traumatic periods of fighting, they had also had extended periods to rest and recover, whereas the young Vietnam veterans had seen enemy fire almost every day of their tour. An additional stressor had been the fact that the enemy in the Vietnam war did not wear a uniform, so the soldiers could not distinguish them from local villagers, and they were thus unable to predict where the next attack would come from. This extended stress had far more damaging and permanent effects on their health.

It was a London cardiologist, Dr Peter Nixon, who in 1979 first elucidated and described the 'Human Function Curve' (Figure 2, below), which depicted graphically the fatiguing stress response.[18]

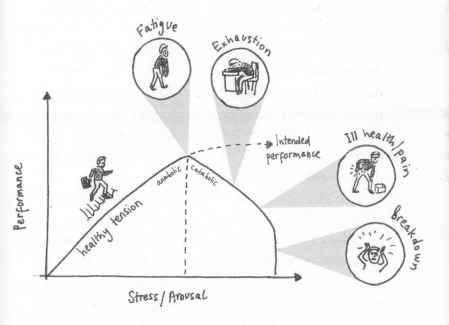

Figure 2: Dr Peter Nixon's Human Function Curve, depicting the fatiguing stress response

What Nixon's graph shows is how the body can absorb, adapt to and cope with ongoing stress for a while – even benefit from it – until a critical inflection point, when, if there is no respite, the system fails, usually resulting in some form of illness. Nixon's work was seminal and has become even more relevant now in the stressful 21st century.

It is important to note that although the curve shape is the same for all of us, the point at which the inflection or collapse occurs will be different. Some people are quite simply better at coping within their environment than others.

GOOD STRESS VERSUS BAD STRESS

In general terms there are two types of stress. The first is *eustress*, which is the sort of exciting, 'on-it' stress that occurs when an individual feels extremely busy but also useful and valued, and excited about the outcome of something. I call this 'benign' stress, because although it may make you tired or bad-tempered, it is short-lived and does not cause illness.

The other type is *distress*. This is the unpleasant or harmful variety which causes illness and disease. I call this sort of stress 'malignant', because it also carries with it the potential and actual ability to cause cancer and heart disease, as well as pain. This is the stress that is cumulative and arises from long-term issues such as an unhappy marriage, childhood trauma or a dead-end job.

A Whitehall study carried out by Professor Michael Marmot, an epidemiologist at UCL, highlighted this in a startling way.[19] It studied 28,000 employees in the civil service from 1967 up to the present day, looking at the social determinants of health, i.e. which are the economic and social conditions that influence individual and group differences in people's health. It discovered that there was a 'status syndrome', where the lower the grade of an employee and the less control they had over their job, the higher their levels of stress and resultant effects on their general health. The further down the hierarchy they were, the higher their levels of disease and mortality rate and the more likely they were to experience pain.

It is not always easy to distinguish good from bad stress, however – and, in some sectors, we are losing our ability to tell the difference. In high-performing, competitive corporate environments, stress has become a dirty word. It is seen as a weakness and so it tends to get 'sucked up' or buried. Even workplace jargon has become unemotive. We don't talk about a 'problem' but a 'challenge' or an 'issue'. More on this later.

As we saw earlier, we *Homo sapiens*, with our hugely developed cerebrums and limbic (mood and emotional) centres, have the ability not only to activate the same flight responses as animals, but also to know when we might need them in the future. We learned to make associations with danger and to predict their likelihood.

As time went on, with our bigger brains, we learned to cook, which meant we could spend less time chewing plants (poor old chimps spend eight hours a day doing it) and more time on social development and cognition. We learned to outwit our predators and prey rather than overpower them. We formed social hierarchies which required sophisticated new behaviour, and we developed emotions to encourage protection and attachment to others. This not only kept us alive but also ensured the propagation of our genes in a new and altruistic way. But with all that came a different kind of stress – psychological stress – because with our increased intellectual capacity came fear, anticipation and anxiety as well as suffering and pain.

Today, when we sit around and worry about mortgages, taxes and public speaking (which for some people is scarier than death), we switch on very similar stress responses to the more physically initiated ones. The problem is that in our modern society we are almost never free of those stressors. The response never stands down; it becomes ever-present, sapping resources. Much like pain, it becomes a habit which is easier to keep with us than to let go of. Research has shown that, when we are continually stressed, a part of the brain known as the amygdala becomes sensitised not just to actual dangers but to small or even potential risks. As a result, we become more anxious and sensitive to threat, and more vulnerable to the very thing that is meant to protect us. We adopt psychological 'crutches' to support the state we are in, either in the form of fear-avoidance behaviours, or by taking stimulants to make us happy and relaxants to keep us calm.

This is the unpleasant, harmful form of stress I mentioned earlier – the one that can cause illness and disease. There is a difference between these two, by the way; illness is a person's subjective experience of their symptoms, while a disease is a definable medical condition. And pain and stress belong in both domains. Basically, if pain and stress continue for long enough, an illness can develop into a real and verifiable disease. So you can feel very unwell, as with the painful and distressing condition known as fibromyalgia, even though there is no detectable evidence of disease. As I explained in Chapter 2, you can have nociception without pain and pain without nociception.

This is an important point because the 'ill', and in most cases 'chronically stressed', rather than the 'diseased', represent a very large number of patients visiting the doctor. Research would suggest that in the USA the number of visits which are for stress-related conditions is as high as 60 to 80 per cent and it looks similar in the UK.[20] However, it is difficult to be very accurate because the studies examine separate symptoms and conditions rather than those specifically related to stress as the cause.

In the UK, most data looks at mental health problems related to stress, a phenomenon which is rising at a terrifying rate; and there is significant overlap of mental health problems with pain. Many of those presenting to their GP will be treated with painkilling drugs, useful or not, or will be referred for expensive tests and scans because the doctors, who are under enormous pressure and have precious little time, will practise 'defensive' medicine and refer them 'just in case'. Most will have nothing abnormal diagnosed and go on to get better anyway. However, the small percentage of these presenting patients who are really sick will not be given the time and attention they need. On average, most British GPs have seven minutes for an appointment.[21] It is worth noting that if the stressed contingent realised their symptoms were a response to their stress and therefore didn't bother going to see their GP about them, the really sick would have much more time with the doctor. Moreover, fewer GPs would be leaving the profession.

○ ○ ○

One of the difficulties in treating people suffering from stress is that we all have different stress thresholds and we all perceive stress differently. For some, stress is external and encapsulates the burden of daily life which is harmful and to be avoided. For others, it is more internal and represents a response inside the body; if we feel anxious about something we say we are 'stressed'. There are high-powered executives for whom it is a status symbol without which they would in some way feel inferior or invalid: the crazily busy, totally stoked man or woman, doing high-stakes deals around the world, meeting fabulous people in fabulous places. Athletes and performers, meanwhile, manage to convert or reframe stress mentally as excitement, readiness, a coming-together of all the elements of their training and a chance to shine and win.

We all have an in-built capacity to cope with stress, with our bodies acting as a buffer. Each time we are tested we can shift the equilibrium a little to absorb the demand. But when those demands become too great or too repetitive, depending on our individual threshold, the balance is disturbed and our well-being is threatened. A situation that is stressful for one person may be benign or even stimulating for another; stress is subjective, like pain – an individual's responses to different stressors relying on their past experience, education, beliefs, personality and genetic make-up. As Hans Selye, the eminent researcher on stress whom I quote at the beginning of this chapter, once said: 'Stress, like beauty, is in the eye of the beholder.' [22]

In 1956, researchers in Montreal looking into nutrition and growth rates in rats made an unexpected discovery about how stress works.[23] During their experiments, it became conspicuously clear that one group of caged rats was not only not thriving but was actually not growing at all, despite being on one of the best diets. It was a PhD student who pointed out the reason why: the rats had been placed within a few feet of a cage containing a cat, which was part of a different study.

The stress of being close to the cat and unable to escape from the cage was inhibiting their growth. When the cage was moved, they quickly caught up. This showed the importance of three factors as contributors to chronic and debilitating stress in the study on rats: an imminent and threatening danger; a constant and unremitting presence of it; and a lack of control over their ability to escape.

Another example which elegantly shows the far-reaching effects of stress (again incidental and unintended) was provided in a study carried out in the 1930s by Dr Elsie Widdowson, a formidable character who pioneered nutritional science and was the first to analyse food and its constituents.[24] After the war she would be tasked with drawing up nutritional programmes for Holocaust survivors.

In her study, Widdowson looked at the effects of different breads on children's growth. Her subjects lived in an orphanage, which was divided into houses run by house mistresses.

Widdowson was puzzled to note that the children in one house failed to grow nearly as quickly as the others. Eventually, a mistress from a different house approached her secretly, and helped shed light on the matter. She explained that the house in which the children were failing to grow was run by a mistress known as 'Dragon-lady', who was notoriously sadistic and mean to the children at mealtimes, castigating and punishing them so that they dreaded eating. It turned out the reason the children were not growing was because of the stress induced by her remonstrations. After 'Dragon-lady' was removed, there was an almost complete recovery in their growth rates.

Stressors can of course be physical (injury, disease, surgery) as well as psychological, but it is the latter that we will focus on here, as psychological stress affects more people more of the time in modern Western and industrialised nations. What's more, it also elicits biological responses which eventually develop into pain, illness and disease. In most, it will produce the symptoms and pain of the 'worried well' or, as psychologist Oliver James so brilliantly coined it 'affluenza'.[25] Sadly, in some, however, it goes on to produce serious conditions such as cancer, diabetes, heart disease and depression (for which I will produce real evidence).

WHEN STRESS AND PAIN COLLIDE

In the UK, pain costs the state more than cancer and diabetes combined,[26] but no one is really talking about it or coming up with answers to treat it. My experience, and that of many other professionals, is that much of this pain is a manifestation of a stress-filled society.

Stress has many strikingly similar traits to pain. Our response to it is very personal and depends on how we assess the demands placed on us and our capacity to cope with them. Psychological stress is as much about how we see the world as about how it really is. And importantly, as with pain, the brain can feel stress without being conscious of it. Subconsciously, too, we can be affected by other people's stress: people who are stressed often exhibit it in their behaviour so that family members or work colleagues pick up on it and feel it themselves.

The 'contagious' nature of stress has been confirmed by research carried out by the US army, which showed that we detect and subliminally respond to the fear and stress hormones (pheromones) secreted by other people; we literally smell their fear.[27]

The evolutionary value of this is clear – it is usful to be able to communicate to the group any gathering or impending threat, and this is particularly pertinent to females and their fertility. In the case of animals, for example, if a new habitat or feeding ground became potentially dangerous, it was not a time to be giving birth or raising offspring; and so the stress response was communicated through the group and resulted in impaired ovarian function and a failure of the eggs to implant. Males in the group would also see a decrease in their libido and sperm count. And that reaction – something that was created by nature to protect the group and allow for agility and mobility in the event of attack – has become in modern times a response that causes enormous angst and misery.

Even though there is no mortal danger, the constant low levels of stress in our society – not helped by the fact that many people are opting to have children much later due to financial pressures – are lowering fertility rates. This in turn causes further stress and anxiety. Indeed, it is now known that such stress activates inflammatory and immune responses in both males and females, which prevent conception. A joint American-British study has shown a correlation between elevated levels of an enzyme associated with stress found in saliva and infertility in women.[28] The study suggests that finding safe ways to alleviate stress may play a role in helping women become pregnant.

And then there is the way in which stress manifests as pain. Many of my patients have expressed the 'pain' of not being able to conceive: not only emotional but physical pain – headaches, and neck and back pain. Some of my female patients also express it as deep pelvic pain, the source of which is chronic tension in their pelvic floor muscles. As one of my very wise tutors used to say: 'This woman's pain is a megaphone for her emotions.' This is just one example of how stress and pain are fundamentally linked and, in many cases, how long-term stress evolves into a physical condition or illness.

From as early as the late 1960s, Dr John Sarno, a rehabilitation specialist, working at the Rusk Institute for Rehabilitation Medicine at New York University, came up with a very interesting theory: that most chronic pain is the result of deep-seated pent-up anger and rage, often originating from childhood.[29]

He believed the patient's subconscious anger was trying

to establish itself consciously as physical pain, in order to distract them from more personal and emotionally painful issues. He discovered that if you could make the patient understand and accept this phenomenon and deal with what was really behind the pain, then the subconscious brain just got back in its box, as it no longer needed to establish itself. If you like, the call from within was being answered. This was particularly the case with hard-working perfectionists, driven by self-imposed pressure that left them feeling stretched to breaking point. Sarno posited the idea, which would later be evidenced by research, that there was a trend in those who had chaotic childhoods, in which they struggled to get control over their unpredictable environments, particularly women, towards producing chronic pain in adulthood.

When Sarno published his book *The Mind-Body Connection* in 1991, it was widely acclaimed – although it was also clear that many in the medical profession, particularly in spinal medicine at the time, wanted his theory to go away as soon as possible, as it threatened to put a spanner in the works of a lucrative industry.

I was lucky enough to train with Sarno and saw him achieve remarkable results with patients who had suffered agonising pain for years. By far the biggest cohort he helped were patients with back pain, which is the most common type of chronic pain. He would famously give them three lectures in order to cure their pain. (I should point out that he did first screen patients by telephone to assess their suitability for his treatment.)

Since Sarno first posited his ideas in the 1960s, medical science has moved forward in leaps and bounds, particularly in the field of imaging and MRI scanning, which is now able to pick up brain activity (known as fMRI). It was Sarno who put the previously poorly described mind/body relationship vis a vis pain on the map, but he was never really appreciated for it. He died in 2017, aged 93, disappointed, I believe, that his ground-breaking work had not been formally recognised and was still regarded as controversial. I think if he could have seen how his ideas are being incorporated into the mainstream today, just a couple of years after his death, he would feel vindicated.

Of course, for many sufferers, the concept that the very real physical pain they feel might have its roots in childhood is hard to take on board. But the fact is that the most consistently identified risk factor in the production of chronic pain is the inability to express emotions, particularly those associated with anger. Repressed anger increases the physiological stress on the person and creates an unnatural biochemical environment in the body. Often other emotional factors are involved, such as hopelessness and lack of social support.

As Gabor Maté has said: 'The person who does not express negative emotion will be isolated even if surrounded by friends, because his real self is not seen. The sense of hopelessness follows from the chronic inability to be true to oneself on the deepest level. Hopelessness leads to helplessness since nothing one can do is perceived as making a difference.' [30]

A Dutch study showed how negative emotions could affect pain.[31] The authors compared female patients who had been diagnosed with fibromyalgia with a group who had no pain. They applied an unchanging painful stimulus to both groups and asked them to grade the pain, firstly when they were thinking about an emotionally sad or angry event, and then when they were thinking about something emotionally neutral. In all cases the pain level reported was higher when the women thought of emotionally negative events, and particularly so in the case of the fibromyalgia sufferers.

Psychological factors such as uncertainty, conflict, lack of control and lack of information are also seen as powerful activators of the stress-response system. The most important of these factors is lack of control – the impact of any stressor depends upon the degree to which it can be controlled, i.e. can the person escape, alter or eliminate the stress or pain? However, many experiments, on both animals and humans, have shown that it is the subject's *perception* of the control they have on their health, rather than their actual degree of control, that has the greatest impact on them.

I have seen in my own clinical practice time and again how important a sense of control is in helping patients deal with chronic pain. A person who believes they are in control of their pain will consistently cope with it better. This has also been demonstrated in an experiment comparing the amount of painkillers required by post-operative patients.[32]

The authors of the study found that those who were put in charge of their own pain medication took far fewer painkillers than those who had them administered. They concluded that this was due to the fact that they didn't have to worry about when they would get the medication from the nurse.

So we can see that the mind and body are constantly striving to return to a state of balance and that they have the capacity to absorb and cope with stresses put upon them and to correct imbalances through various adaptive compensating mechanisms. Hippocrates made this point way back in the 5th century BC when he taught that disease is not only suffering or pain (*pathos*) but also toil (*ponos*); the fight of the body to restore itself to normal. These processes are better understood now. And understanding them, as well as being able to recognise when they are under strain and where that strain comes from, is the answer to relieving the suffering of many.

This is all good news. Because, by changing how we view the world, learning to understand stress and when we are subject to it, we can alter our susceptibility to it and its most frequent outcome – pain.

On the page opposite is a working pictorial representation of how I assess a patient's situation with respect to their pain and the contributing stressors affecting their system. I have it on my desk and in my mind's eye while taking a history. Remember the bio-psycho-social model we discussed in Chapter 1? Well, the same interlocking rings are relevant to both the pain and stress factors in a patient's life. And, if we superimpose the two, we end up with a model by which to assess which factors are key to that person in terms of where their pain and stress collide, and which factors are less relevant – i.e. is the pain/stress coming mostly from the psychological sphere? Or is it more socially motivated? Which area do we need to work on to bring them back into balance?

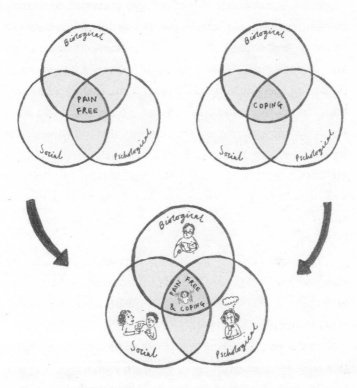

Figure 3: The bio-psycho-social model of pain and stress factors
and how they interlock

CASE HISTORY: LUCY

It is here that I want to introduce you to Lucy, who presented with painful symptoms that were ultimately the
result of a long-term stress response.

79

Lucy was 34 and a successful executive in a small media firm which employed 100 people. She had been promoted to senior management and reported directly to the CEO, Michael.

Lucy was engaged to be married and arrangements had begun for the wedding. She was conscientious and something of a perfectionist. She generally over-worried about life but that also made her good at her job.

She came to see me because she had done the rounds of therapists and surgeons for ongoing head-aches, neck and facial pain, and tinnitus. She frequently experienced pins and needles in her face and hands. She felt foggy-brained most of the time and her sleep was poor. Her anxiety was worsened by the fact that no one seemed to be able to help her or identify the source of the problem. She was convinced she had multiple scle-rosis and had googled a number of her symptoms, which only worried her more.

Various doctors had begun to imply that she was sim-ply neurotic because all of her scans were normal. In fact, the more they imaged her, the more concerned she became.

From her very first appointment, it was obvious that Lucy suffered with hyperventilation (breathing too shal-lowly and rapidly) and tended to hold her breath for extended periods. When she did take a breath, she used her neck, shoulder and chest muscles all the time, acting against gravity and wasting energy. She looked washed out and tired and her hands were pale and cold. She also sweated a lot from her armpits, which made her feel self-conscious at work, so she never took her suit jacket off. She had lost her confidence and had become very self-critical, and dreaded presenting to colleagues as she got tongue-tied and forgot details. She had experienced a decrease in her libido, which worried her further because she was hoping to get pregnant soon after the wedding.

In short, her outlook on life had become very negative and she was concerned she was becoming depressed. She had fought low moods as a teenager but thought that she had kicked them. She had also recently put on weight around her belly and she just couldn't shift it.

I started by reassuring Lucy that all was not lost and that I was pretty sure she not only did not have MS but that the source and cure for the problem was fairly simple.

I got her to lie on the examination couch and taught her how to breathe from her diaphragm – by asking her to expand and contract her belly and not her chest as she breathed. Immediately, the tight and tender muscles in her shoulders and chest relaxed, and she became less clammy.

I explained how her posture had changed due to the breathing dysfunction and that her postural muscles never rested and were full of painful trigger points. Many of these points were in her jaw and neck muscles, and were causing her headaches.

I asked her to wear a breathing monitor for a week

which would 'speak' to her phone and track her breathing. It would also buzz at her when it caught her holding her breath or breathing erratically. At her next appointment, when we looked at the tracking app, we discovered that Lucy regularly went into erratic breathing and, at a specific time (3pm) on specific days (Tuesday and Thursday), markedly held her breath. I asked Lucy what it was that she was doing at this time that stressed her so.

She was surprised when she realised that the 3 o'clock slot was a twice-weekly catch-up meeting with her boss, Michael. I asked her how she felt about her relationship with him, and she admitted that she found him difficult and volatile and that he seemed to shut her down when she was being creative or wanted to take a lead on something. He also tended to undermine her in front of junior colleagues. We went back over her childhood and discovered that Lucy's father had been an alcoholic. When he was drinking he was volatile and she and her siblings would tiptoe around him, trying not to antagonise him. Her mother had always been timid and submissive with him and implored them not to upset him. As a result, Lucy had always dreaded and avoided confrontation.

I suggested to Lucy that elements of Michael's behaviour might remind her of her father and that she was struggling to assert herself with him. She agreed that this was a distinct possibility. I proposed some strategies to help her move forward with him, including suggesting to him that they had a drink outside work to discuss their relationship issues. Bravely, Lucy did this and it was a great success. Michael admitted that he felt threatened by her as she was clearly capable and more creative than he was. By discussing her feelings with him, Lucy had encouraged him to open up. Over the next month, the improvement in their working relationship, and the general atmosphere in the office, was evident to all concerned.

Most importantly, the rest of Lucy's symptoms faded away. This is not to say that she would not face stressful situations in the future, but she now had all the tools to treat herself, and could recognise when a confrontation needed to be broached. The fear and dread involved in doing so also waned with practice. Her confidence grew. Equally gratifying for her was that the corset of fat that had developed around her middle – the classic fat distribution of long-term cortisol secretion which causes the body to store fat in this way – disappeared without her needing to diet. Lucy's body had been releasing the hormone cortisol into her system due to the long-term stress she had been under. As we will find out later, there are a number of processes that cortisol changes, including how and where we deposit fat.

I suggested to Lucy that she seek professional help from a psychologist to help her deal further with the issues around her difficult childhood and the anger she had towards her father. For although we had succeeded for now in ridding her of her pain, I was concerned that it would either re-present itself or create a problem somewhere else. She has continued to use the breathing device as it helps her know when she is shifting into a stressed state and it keeps her calm.

CHAPTER 4

HOW STRESS MAKES US HURT

'He who fears he shall suffer, already
suffers what he fears.'
– Montaigne

Any one of us can succumb to illness and pain at any time.
We then have a choice: we can take a passive role, allowing
the doctor to take authority, or we can decide to be actively
and knowledgeably involved in our own care – which
implies taking a more holistic approach: i.e. why have I
developed this pain? How is it going to affect my life? How
do I feel about it? It is enormously empowering to realise
that one is not a passenger but a co-driver on the route
to health. And to do this we need to get to grips with the
link between psychology, emotion and physiology because
understanding this gives us a vital tool for the process of
our recovery.

As Dr Gabor Maté says, it is important to understand
that how you *feel* is the summation of all your bodily

processes: 'Physiologically, emotions are themselves electrical, chemical and hormonal discharges of the human nervous system. Emotions influence – and are influenced by – the functioning of our major organs, the integrity of our immune defences and the workings of many circulating biological substances that help govern the body's physical states.' [33]

In this chapter, I hope to convince you or at least tweak your curiosity enough to make you consider deeply some fascinating truths around human behaviour: namely, how we respond to stress and how it makes us ill. This is a chapter about 'mind over disease' and the connections between the brain and immune system which mediate our health. I will show you that our mental and physical states are inextricably linked, and that stress and other psychological factors not only cause pain but also often alter our vulnerability to bacterial and viral infections as well as cancer, heart disease and diabetes.

In the words of the celebrated neuroscientist and pharmacologist, Professor Candace Pert: 'It is this problem of unhealed feeling, the accumulation of bruised and broken emotions that most people stagger under without ever saying a word, that the mainstream medical model is least effective in dealing with.' [34]

Most importantly, I want you to consider that what is going on with your health, physical or mental, may be down to something, or things, you have not yet thought about. You may need to address other possible contributing elements, not just the obvious symptoms. Accepting the possibility that life and all that it throws at you is as much a cause of your pain as an injury or condition is the first step to sorting it out.

○ ○ ○

Dr Hans Kraus was the New York physician who famously treated and cured US President John F Kennedy's spinal pain after years of failed attempts by other doctors. Kraus discovered that, though young and lean in physique, JFK was muscularly as weak as a kitten and as stiff as a board, and so he devised an intense programme of flexibility and strengthening exercises for him.

Having completed this regime, JFK was almost pain-free, and even able to play golf again. Kraus had identified a condition he termed 'muscle tension syndrome', which he said existed predominantly in people who were exposed to significant and constant levels of stress.

In his book *Backache, Stress and Tension*, Kraus explained where this tension came from: 'Your muscles, your mind, your heart and all your organs prepare to act, but you do nothing… You may wish to fight, you may wish to flee, but modern civilisation prevents you from carrying out your natural impulses… You race your engines without going anywhere.' [35]

I have noticed in my own practice that the paradoxical relationship between inactivity (particularly in those in corporate sedentary jobs) and mental stress embodies this idea exactly. The stress response wants us to act but – stuck to our seats – we constantly repress what we feel, or rather what society feels, would be an inappropriate response physically.

My mentor, Dr John Sarno, whom I mentioned in the

previous chapter, embraced the Kraus approach and developed the idea still further. He found that, although many patients responded to an exercise programme, this did not resolve all their issues. And he noticed that, although their pain might improve initially, the symptoms would often return or simply move and manifest themselves somewhere else in the body. He quickly saw a pattern develop in many of his patients, that their pain was a manifestation of repressed emotional turmoil and that this resulted in oxygen deprivation and a build-up of waste products from metabolism, which was responsible for the muscle tension and neurological irritation.

This realm of interconnectedness between the psychological processes, the hormonal glands and the immune systems that regulate our behaviour and physiological balance is the subject of a fascinating area of study known as psycho-neuroendocrine-immunology, or PNI.

You will remember, from earlier chapters, the idea of nociception: that is, the sensory input from the body which is sent to the brain for assessment and analysis (bottom-up)? And you will remember that pain only occurs when the brain decides to recognise the information it receives from nociception (top-down)? Well, PNI is the system that the brain mobilises to *carry out a response* to all of the stuff it has analysed and decided needs action. The psycho- bit represents the cognitive element through which we decide what to do; the neuroendocrine- is the linked system of nerves and hormones which communicate a call to action and the specific response in different tissues and organs. The -immunology bit refers to the myriad responses in the immune system to set off inflammation if there is a need to heal, as well as the specialist cells needed to fight any infection which gets into the body as a result.

There is now consistent and growing evidence from thousands of scientific studies for a connection between life events, personality type, stress and the psychological causes of subsequent pain, disease and even malignancy.[36] These life events don't need to be extreme or traumatic; the cumulative effect of life's mundane trials and tribulations can also have an impact on health over time. The diseases of multiple sclerosis and rheumatoid arthritis are good examples of conditions where stressful childhood parental relationships, life adversity or traumatic events either just before the onset of the disease or as a causative agent in its symptom exacerbation have been strongly linked. The common process involved in these conditions is inappropriate persistent inflammation in tissues causing long-term damage.

As early as 1939, John Scott Haldane, a British physiologist, had a hunch about the involvement of psychological factors in disease and wrote: 'The commonest cause of gastritis, an inflamed and irritable stomach, is worry and anxiety. I had it for 15 years and then I read Lenin on Society and how to cure it. Since then I am cured.' [37]

Food for thought! (Though reading Lenin is not something I regularly prescribe for my patients.)

○ ○ ○

PNI is essentially a bodily communication system in which all the components – our thoughts, emotions, immune system and hormones – are linked by a network of two-way pathways, with one agenda: to ensure our survival and reproduction and the propagation of our genes. These connections allow the system to recognise both internal and external threats and respond with appropriate behaviour and biochemical reactions to maximise safety at as little cost as possible. This 'super-system' is hardwired together by the nervous system. Even the glandular and immune centres (e.g. bone marrow, thyroid and thymus glands), which were once thought to be acted on only by hormones, are extensively supplied by nerves. Within the nervous system there are many different types of neurones which serve different functions. Some simply connect other nerves, some feed, nourish and repair them, and some monitor the need for change and action it locally if necessary. But they all serve to facilitate the communication between all of the four systems of the PNI, whether it is to increase or decrease a response or just feed back to the brain on the current state of things as to how much to respond (See figure 4 overleaf).

So, the amazing news is that the brain can talk to and monitor every system in the body… and, likewise, each of the hormones and immune cells can exert their own influence on the brain. The chemicals produced by all these systems attach to receptors on brain cells, thereby directly affecting our behaviour.

Almost all cells, by the way, have receptors on their surfaces for molecules coming from the brain – this is how the brain communicates directly with the immune system and this is why any short- or long-term stimulus which acts on any part of the PNI system is felt by every other part to some degree. The stressor exerts an effect on us which causes a shift or response in the entire system. The chatter is passed down the line to every cell, regardless of its primary function. Think of the cells as being like people on a crowded tube train, everyone jostling and adjusting as one more passenger gets on. A good example of this is the white blood cells, which are the main defenders of the immune system against invaders or disease and can produce almost all the same hormones and neurotransmitters that the brain cells can. They can even produce the mood-altering and pain-relieving chemicals known as endorphins – our own happy pills. On the downside these white blood cells can produce their own chemicals (cytokines) which in the brain exert their effect as pain and depression, and in the joints as pain and swelling. The effects can be felt anywhere in the body – not just at the site of the infection.

So, we can see that there is a big 'conversation' going on throughout the body via a super-system of messengers using what could almost be described as a 'molecular language'.

We have all experienced the sensation of being exposed to a brief episode of stress such as a near-miss with another car. We get the 'prickly armpit' sensation, rapid pulse and sweaty palms that are due to a hormone we are all familiar with: adrenaline. This is produced in the adrenal glands, located just above the kidneys.

All the cognitive and emotional centres within the brain that detect danger and threat communicate with the rest of the body through one hub called the hypothalamus, a region deep in the brain, just above the pituitary gland. And when we perceive immediate danger or fear, signals are sent via the hypothalamus, using adrenaline.

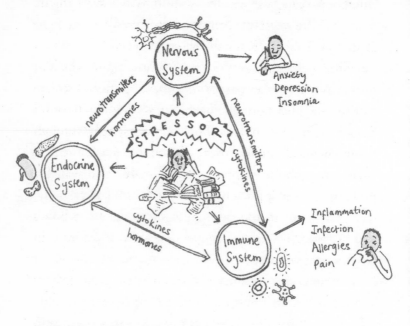

Figure 4: The PNI system, which connects our emotions, thoughts, hormones and immune system.

Adrenaline acts on a part of the nervous system called the autonomic nervous system, which has two distinct parts: the sympathetic system, which governs our immediate 'fight or flight' response; and the parasympathetic system, which governs our 'rest and digest' functions. In an ideal world, most of the time we should be in the zen-like parasympathetic domain: relaxed, ruminating, digesting, making love and going about our daily activities, and only nudging into the sympathetic zone occasionally when roused.

However, due to the stresses of our modern lives now, and any that we may have experienced in our formative childhood years, we tend to shift into the sympathetic domain. Here we sit in a constant state of readiness to fight or to run. This is OK for the short term but if it goes on too long, messages get sent to the hypothalamus, which in turn activates another part of the adrenal glands to secrete cortisol, the uber-hormone of the stress response. Cortisol has a huge number of effects on the PNI system, through many chemical and electrical messengers. Its immediate effect is to mobilise energy systems to make them available for survival. And it acts on almost every tissue of the body; from the brain to the immune system and from bones to intestines. Despite there being a general increase in immune activity during stress, cortisol's immediate effect is to dampen the stress reaction, keeping immune activity within safe levels. The stress response can be seen not only as the body's reaction to threat but also as its attempt to maintain stability and homeostasis. The body is held, if you like, in a state of physiologically controlled panic.

It was Dr Hans Selye who first described how the biology of stress affected three types of tissue or organs: in the hormonal system (enlarged adrenal glands); in the immune system (spleen, thymus and lymph glands); and in the digestive system (intestinal lining). In one of his first studies, rats exposed to stress for long periods showed enlarged adrenals, shrunken lymph nodes and ulcerated intestines.[38] This would explain why so many stress sufferers present with stomach and intestinal problems and ulcers.

The most pertinent element of the cortisol response for our purposes, as we think about chronic pain, is its effect on inflammation.

In a study he conducted at Carnegie Mellon University,

Professor Sheldon Cohen showed that chronic psycholog-ical stress is associated with the body losing its ability to regulate the inflammatory response, because the immune cells in the tissues become insensitive to cortisol.[39] (Some practitioners have begun to refer to this state as adrenal fatigue, although that remains a controversial diagnosis.) Cohen's was a major finding as it solved a conundrum that the medical profession had struggled with for some time: namely, if cortisol inhibited the inflammatory response – indeed, cortisol injections have been used for many years to ease inflamed and painful joints – how could it also stimulate it? Cohen discovered that the acute short-term effects of cortisol are indeed *anti*-inflammatory but that with prolonged secretion the effect is lost.

He went on to show that the effects of psychological stress on the body's ability to regulate inflammation can promote the development and progression of diseases such as joint disease and autoimmune conditions such as rheumatoid arthritis, which predominantly manifest in the inflammatory response and the failure to recognise 'self' – the so-called 'friendly fire' effect. Cohen observed that when cortisol is not able to serve its regulatory function, inflammation can get out of control. Such inflammation can affect a multitude of tissues, most particularly the linings of the joints and the spine, and the stomach and digestive system.

New and exciting research has shown that the chemicals I mentioned earlier, cytokines, which are actively involved in the inflammatory stress response, can also cross what is known as the blood–brain barrier, which was previ-ously thought impossible, as is elegantly described by Dr

Edward Bullmore in his book *The Inflamed Mind*.[40] It is now believed that cytokines which get through the specialist cells (endothelial cells) lining the small blood vessels of the brain can trigger inflammation in the brain and that this may be the source of many forms of depression and possibly even dementia. This finding has raised many new questions, for example whether people suffering with painful arthritis are depressed simply because of the pain or whether in fact depression is part of the inflammatory process affecting the sensitive neural tissues.

The details are still uncertain but people who are depressed show an array of immunological changes, even without other illness being present. Equally, people who have a lot of inflammation in their bodies, such as rheumatoid arthritis, frequently report depression as well as higher levels of pain.

Cohen, in his research, also showed that people who were exposed to a prolonged stressful event and who were therefore unable to control the inflammatory response were much more likely to succumb to a cold virus. He demonstrated that stress has an impact on heart disease and asthma, because these conditions are also inflammation-based.

In 2013, a joint study carried out by several US universities, led by UCLA and Ohio State, found that individuals who had chronic exposure to adverse environments (bereavement, social isolation and low socio-economic status) showed increased inflammation in their bodies[41] – that their sympathetic nervous system stimulated their bone marrow to produce immature pro-inflammatory cells and that this inflammation was capable of causing pain at multiple sites. Furthermore, it was shown to inhibit the production of genes designed to mount an immune response to viruses. Hence many sufferers of cold sores (which are caused by a herpes simplex virus) report that they develop a sore only when they are stressed or run down. The dip in the immune system function allows the virus to activate itself. Shingles, another herpes virus, follows a similar pattern. These viruses which live within us permanently, are suppressed by a healthy immune system until we are stressed either by our environment or by another infection, 'distracting' the immune system from it.

Obesity is another cause of stress on our systems that results in inflammation. We now know that people who are significantly overweight and who as a result produce adipose tissue (a form of body fat) have increased levels of inflammation in their bodies. Researchers have shown that an overload of fat in our bodies damages the *mitochondria*, the 'power generators' in our cells, which are responsible for providing energy for metabolism.[42] The body then mounts an immune response to repair or break down the damaged mitochondria. And this leads to inflammation in the tissues, which causes joint pain and arthritis, and inflammation of the blood vessel walls, which results in atherosclerosis, a cause of stroke and heart disease.

If that weren't enough to convince you of the dangers of stress, there is also now evidence that a vicious cycle can develop between obesity and cortisol. Cortisol is known to increase the absorption of fat when we are stressed and classically redistributes it around and inside the abdomen. When going through stressful periods, even slim people who do not overeat can discover that they have fat around their middles which they cannot shift. This is the most serious type of weight gain as it is the most detrimental to health. It is why the medical profession has started using the hip-to-waist ratio (which involves dividing the circumference of your waist by that of your hips) rather than Body Mass Index to measure obesity.

So we can see how, paradoxically, a biochemical system designed to preserve life becomes a major cause of pain and illness. In the short term, this mechanism is extremely effective in the emergencies it was designed to protect us from. But if triggered for prolonged periods and without remission, it produces permanent damage and long-lasting pain. Chronically stimulated, adrenaline raises blood pressure and damages the heart, while cortisol impairs the immune system and damages tissue.

The awkward truth here is that science is now proving that the 'H' word, *holism* (treating the whole person, taking into account medical and social factors, rather than just the symptoms of disease) is the way forward. Holistic medicine has become associated with quackery, snake oil and wooden beads, but in many ways it resembles how the old-school avuncular physicians approached the patient's story. With fewer diagnostic tests at their disposal, country GPs (think of the TV series *Dr Finlay's Casebook* if you are old enough) viewed patients within the context of their environment and used as much life wisdom to treat them as medical knowledge. They honed their bedside manner with the use of time-honoured clinical skills which reassured their patients.

With a move towards a symptom-based reductionist philosophy of tests and imaging, driven by the infiltration of profit-obsessed pharmaceutical and biotech companies into hospitals, medical schools and universities, the old-style holistic principles have long been sidelined and are now applied only by alternative healing practitioners.

Gratifyingly, and in my own practice lifetime, we are beginning to see a swing back towards a more 360-degree view of illness and disease – though using new terms such as 'functional' or 'integrated' medicine, rather than the 'H' word. And this, I hope, is going to change the whole approach to the treatment of pain.

CASE HISTORY: MAX

Twenty-year-old Max came to see me with his mother. His family is well-off and have lived all over the world. Max had been to the best schools, and he emphasised the fact that he was now doing a psychology degree, as if to warn me off indulging in any psychobabble. At several stages he had been at boarding school and thus living apart from his parents, who are now separated. The tension between Max and his mother was palpable, and he barely looked at either her or me as he related his tale. He had a constant air of angry petulance and sighed or held his breath every few seconds. He referred to his mother for details he clearly knew himself and was on edge constantly. It was obvious that he was treated as the 'sickly child that needed to be fixed'. He sweated nervously and had clammy palms when we shook hands. He was tall and very lean, and from the way he sat, folded his arms and fidgeted, I could see he was hypermobile (double-jointed). He smelt strongly of tobacco and the scent of marijuana emanated from every pore. He had rowed competitively at school and university.

Max had a set of musculoskeletal symptoms that he couldn't cope with any more. He had head, neck and back pain and he always felt twisted physically. Indeed, one practitioner had told him that his symptoms were all down to scoliosis, being born with a twisted spine. Additionally, he was light-headed and struggled to sleep and concentrate. He frequently had palpitations.

Max had seen a multitude of practitioners, both conventional and alternative, but none had managed to get to the bottom of his issues and his parents had spent a fortune on tests and imaging.

He was understandably sceptical as to whether I would be able to help him. His mother wanted to stay in the room even for his examination. Max did not actually protest but it was clear he would rather she was not there, particularly as I asked him to undress so I could examine him. It was almost as if he knew it was inappropriate that she should stay but he wanted her to be there all the same.

When I examined his back, I saw he had a marginal 'S' bend curve in his spine, of only a few degrees. On my computer, I showed Max a picture of another patient's anonymised X-ray, which had a dramatic scoliosis of 52 degrees. He drew in his breath and said, 'Will I end up like that? She must be in agony!' I explained that she wasn't actually, and never had been, despite how impressively twisted she was. This went some way to reassuring him, but I also asked him: 'If she isn't in pain, how come you are, with such a small curve?'

He thought about this for a moment and raised his eyebrows quizzically. I told him that, despite all the things reported on MRI and X-ray, his curve had almost nothing to do with the pain he complained of. I explained that a lot of the asymmetrical muscle tension on the left-hand side of his low back was in fact due to years of rowing with one oar on the same side. Over the period of ten years that he had been competing, he had developed a shortened pattern in the muscles on one side because it had never been addressed. This was further reflected in the very small muscles at the base of his skull, on the opposite side, where he had been compensating through his neck to keep his eyes on horizontal. All of this was exacerbated by the deep intrinsic muscle tension that he constantly experienced, primarily due to his 'Type A' perfectionist and controlling character, and his all-round 'high-performance' upbringing. Max had no control over his current state and that bothered him too. He had never been allowed to relax or really enjoy life, because it was always about competing either academically or in the sporting arena or even within his own family, where success was expected and praised.

During the little time he spent with his parents, he would always seek their approval and affirmation by impressing them. Throughout his schooling he had always been a survivor and had seemed very resilient but he was not able to express himself emotionally, nor did he really know how he felt. All he knew was that he had to be in a constant state of readiness.

I explained to Max that he was hypermobile in many of his joints and soft tissues and this meant that his muscles had to work harder to fight against gravity and maintain his posture. This would make his muscles ache and cause him pain.

He was surprised when I asked, 'Do you find that you need to move to think? That sitting still is always a problem for you and that you fidget in cinemas and tap your foot?'

His eyes almost welled up in relief that someone finally understood him. His gaze, which had previously flitted around the room, now fixed me intently. I went on to explain to him that it was clear from the way he fired his core muscles that he had not learned to crawl properly as a child – a major motor coordination developmental milestone.

Indeed, his mother confirmed that he'd gone straight to walking but had needed a lot of help. I suspected that although he had no problems with coordination in real terms, he had always been slightly clumsy and always lacked the speed, strength and agility that many of his friends had. That is why he had taken up rowing: as a sport, it does not require multi-skilled tasks. The pressure – and his ultimate failure – to be in the other 'A' sports teams had pushed him towards it.

The first thing to do with Max was to try to teach him to cope with his stress regarding his performance and show him that when he relaxed his muscles, he not only felt less twisted but also in less pain, and that his mind would calm and he would sleep better. I asked him to stop smoking marijuana as it is a drug of withdrawal and as such was preventing him from engaging in what he needed to do to get better. We could teach him to switch off by other means. I also asked him to avoid caffeine and nicotine for three months as we tried to calm his nervous system down.

I gave him my Bakpro tools – a specialist kit for pain relief I have developed[43] – to help him release the painful trigger points that had developed in his muscles at multiple sites. This would not only help him reduce and eventually eliminate his pain but also teach him that he had better control over his condition than he thought. Over the next few sessions, I asked his mother not to come with him; this removed the gag on him talking about his family life and the pressure involved. I manipulated and mobilised all his spinal restrictions, which quickly got rid of his headaches, and taught him exercises to release the asymmetry in his muscles.

At our subsequent appointments, Max no longer had clammy hands and he did not sweat so profusely. He was palpably calmer, and his posture was relaxed. The colour had returned to his face due to the improved oxygenation of his tissues now that he did not hyperventilate. For the first time in some years, he discovered the benefits and delights of a good night's sleep and was more able to concentrate on his work. He had found it surprisingly easy to give up smoking dope now that life was better.

Perhaps most gratifyingly, Max now had a delightful girlfriend whom he brought to meet me one day. She said she had always liked Max in class, but he was always so 'wired' and intense. He always moaned about his health. She noticed that one day something seemed to change in him, and she liked it. So she said yes when he asked her out.

CHAPTER 5

THE SILENT EPIDEMIC

'We are more often frightened than hurt; and we suffer more from imagination than from reality.'
– Lucius Annaeus Seneca

We live in a world where chronic pain is becoming increasingly normal. In the UK, between a third and a half of adults report that they live with some sort of chronic pain. For the over 75s, that number is closer to two thirds.

One big study, Pain in Europe (PIE), which involved 46,000 subjects, showed that one in five adults experienced persistent pain and one in three households had someone in chronic pain.[44] Interestingly, this result was split between the sexes pretty evenly, but more women present to clinics (64 per cent). Pain services need to do more to engage men in confronting their issues and getting help. Of the total number in the study, 80 per cent of subjects presented with musculoskeletal pain, predominantly in the back.

Despite this apparently even split in the sexes, further

research shows that women have the rougher time of it. Four to five times more women than men suffer from chronic pain conditions that afflict both sexes, such as fibromyalgia, migraine and IBS. They will also report greater pain than men with the same illness. This has been confirmed by large global studies in 2008, 2009 and 2012.[45]

Research has shown that women have a lower pain threshold; although they are more used to feeling pain (menstruation, childbirth), in research their ratings of the unpleasantness of pain are always higher than those of men.[46] Interestingly, women are also less sensitive to some painkillers than men. The natural assumption might be that there are hormonal differences which are responsible for the difference in sensitivity. However, extensive research into this area has shown almost no relationship between hormonal changes and pain.[47] The only small correlation was that existing pain can go up at different stages of women's menstrual cycles.

There is growing evidence that women have a more intense emotional response to pain than men. Studies have shown that they tend to accumulate pain experiences over time – something known as *temporal summation* – and that this is partly because they express greater anxiety over pain. Researchers at UCLA, the University of Maryland and Harvard Medical School found that, on fMRI scanners, many of the same brain areas light up for men and women, but in women, the limbic system, which attaches emotion to pain, is also switched on, whereas in men, it's the cognitive or analytic regions (prefrontal cortex) that are activated.[48] Thus it appears that women's pain is heightened by a greater association between pain and suffering, and a perception of pain as a threat.

The evolutionists among us would posit that this is because of the traditional role of woman as carer and protector: anything that posed a threat to her also posed a threat to the survival of her offspring. Thus she was primed to attach greater fear and anxiety to events.

We also now know that some people are susceptible to an inherited predisposition (i.e. it's in your genes) to developing persistent pain. A good way to study this phenomenon is by looking at sets of identical twins, as they share the same genetic material. Three major studies carried out in the UK and Scandinavia found that in back and neck pain, susceptibility ran from 30 to 76 per cent. The Finns found that fibromyalgia was 51 per cent inherited.[49] It was a similar figure for migraine and osteoarthritis.

But this raises an interesting question: why don't all identical twins with the susceptibility or predisposition get the illness? Often one twin will suffer and the other won't. The answer is being increasingly explained by *epigenetics*, 'genetic control by factors other than an individual's DNA sequence'. This means that some genes are only expressed according to the environmental stimuli that a person is exposed to. Molecules called histones, deep within our genetic material, determine which genes are activated. The changes that one individual makes can be passed down to the next generation; but the changes are dependent on the environment of the individual. Research at the University of Texas has shown that epigenetic changes that occur in response to inflammation or nerve injury can lead to persistent pain as they alter pain-modulating pathways.[50] Adaptation works both ways, so the message is: don't let your genes dictate you, dictate them!

Clearly, we all feel pain differently, depending on our life experience, social environment and genetic make-up, and in the treatment of chronic pain, we practitioners need to be aware of this, and to understand the context of the pain and its dynamic in order to have any chance of healing it. Instead of seeing it as a bunch of symptoms that are present because of a neurological condition, we need to hear the patient's story, understand the environment in which it developed and consider the many subtle and subliminal types of stressors that exert their effect on an almost daily basis. Everything that has fed into that pain state is important.

Practitioners like myself also need to be aware that living with chronic pain causes other symptoms as well, such as depression. If you have suffered with intense pain for a long time, your brain will assume this is the state in which you are going to have to live from now on. As a result, it will begin to shed the neural pathways and synapses that normally give you pain-free pleasure and reinforce the synapses and networks that relate to fear and despair.

In this chapter I want to look at this all-important context of pain – the myriad elements in our environment which are causing us stress and why they are increasing in our modern world. As Dr Hans Selye pointed out, most of the stressors in the lives of human beings today are emotional. And yet we have lost touch with the gut feelings designed to be our warning system. We keep ourselves in physiologically stressful situations, with very little, if any, awareness of distress.

Just like the laboratory rats we talked about in Chapter

3, people find themselves trapped in lifestyles and emotional patterns that are hostile to their health. The physiology of stress eats away at us, not because it is no longer necessary but because we no longer have the ability to recognise its signals.

That emotional causes of the stress response can be life-threatening is nowhere better exemplified than in the very real phenomenon of 'dying of a broken heart'. This is known medically as Takotsubo syndrome and happens when a stressful event causes a rush of adrenaline to flood the heart. The left ventricle of the heart swells and adopts the shape of an ancient Japanese octopus pot (from which it gets its name) and causes heart failure. It is usually temporary but if not recognised can be fatal. It is commonly associated with sudden bereavement.

The research literature repeatedly identifies three key factors that lead to stress: uncertainty, lack of information and loss of control. All three of these factors are usually present in the lives of people with chronic pain – many of whom realise that it is the illusion of control that has masked the reasons for many of their decisions and behaviour. And it is often pain or disease that shatters that illusion of control later.

A good but extreme example of where a perceived loss of control and a need for information brings on pain, is the condition we now call post-traumatic stress disorder (PTSD). It is an example of where a cyclical stress response can become a living hell of fear, anxiety and pain. PTSD was first recognised during the First World War, when it was known as 'shellshock'. The soldiers showed no signs of physical injury but exhibited extreme nervousness, muscle spasms, bodily pain, headaches, fits and outbursts of temper and aggression. These symptoms were the result of their normal stress responses becoming numbed, due to unrelenting trauma. The protective effect of cortisol released in the bloodstream was lost and their bodies were exposed to the continued secretion of adrenaline and the resultant constant arousal of the nervous system.

As a consequence, they would suffer flashbacks and nightmares and behave erratically and violently, but at the same time feel cut off from their emotions and unable to speak about what they were doing or feeling. It was Sigmund Freud who first properly elucidated the nature of what was going on psychologically.[51] It all seemed to stem from an effort to seek a degree of control over their experiences. Freud realised that the patient's unconscious mind was constantly returning him to past traumas, both through dreams and while under hypnosis. He concluded that people developed a compulsion to repeat painful experiences, through dreams and flashbacks, in an attempt to switch from the status of passive victims to that of active instigators. It seems that the repetition of painful experiences, this 'compulsion to repeat', to 'restore an earlier state of things', allows us to attain control over them, a conclusion that has been confirmed by modern neuroscience. In his book *Nervous States*, political economist and sociologist William Davies writes: 'The compulsion to repeat teaches us that the essence of trauma is not pain, but the acute disempowerment that leaves one vulnerable to pain even if just as a possibility.' [52]

○ ○ ○

Stressors can appear in our lives as early as childhood, so that many chronic pains, illnesses and autoimmune conditions that emerge in adulthood are not sudden new developments but the culmination of a lifelong process. Even our families, no matter how happy and stable they may seem, can be a source of early angst and are influential in our development emotionally. As Zadie Smith says in her book of essays, *Feel Free*: 'Every family home is an emotionally violent place, full of suppressed rage, struck through with profound individual disappointments. It is in the nature of the beast that no one gets out of the family unit with everything they want.' [53]

Or as the stand-up comedian Jerry Seinfeld puts it: 'There's no such thing as fun for all the family.'

It is worth mentioning some sociological factors here. At the time of writing, the UK is embroiled in Brexit. Don't worry: I am not going into the political whys and wherefores of the whole process – I have no expertise in that area – it is the effect it is having on all our lives that I am interested in: that of uncertainty, stemming from the realisation that we cannot possibly predict with any accuracy how life might change, because we simply have never done it before.

Interestingly, during the period of negotiations, more patients than ever were coming into my clinic with entirely stress-induced symptoms, evident in their breathing patterns and the painful muscle problems they presented with. There was no structural or organic defect or disease to be found, but the symptoms (pain, dizziness, pins and needles and feeling foggy-brained) were real. Some of my patients were experiencing flare-ups of old problems because the cortisol circulating around their bodies had reignited the inflammatory response in their joints. Worry and anxiety also reduce the threshold at which pain is established in the brain. Uncertainty is a danger to us and so pain is established to alert and protect us. This is a good example of where the biological (inflammation/immune response) and the psychological domains intersect.

Or, as William Davies has put it: 'Pain carves a path directly between the realms of mind and body, engulfing us in a psychosomatic fashion.'[54]

However, we have to be careful how we approach the subject of psychosomatic pain, because if we perceive it to be due in its entirety to our environment, about which we feel powerless, then we may feel that there is little we can do to reduce the reality or severity of it. In this situation, 'positive thinking', so often used in therapy, is simply denial. We need to come up with strategies to address the pain and at the same time be less affected by our environment.

In these modern times of seemingly constant stress, we tend to look for chemical 'crutches' to help us cope. The low mood and uncertain emotions induced by our lives lower the level of dopamine in our brains. Dopamine is the neurotransmitter chemical we produce naturally in response to things that make us happy. We love dopamine because it makes us feel at one with the world and it lowers our sense of unhappiness. But in making us happier, it also increases our sense of 'wanting' and so becomes addictive in higher concentrations. It acts on many centres in the brain, but most importantly it controls our motivation to do things. Without realising it, we reach for things that stimulate it in us when it is low, then we get addicted to the higher levels that other chemicals can artificially induce. We become dopamine addicts.

Coffee is the most obvious one, and as a result a rash of coffee shops has broken out in high streets all over the world. Caffeine is known to be a stimulant of serotonin and dopamine (both happy chemicals) and briefly raises our depleted sources of them. The morning double espresso kick-starts our day after a poor night's sleep, but, ironically, the reason for the restless night is the large amounts of coffee we drank the day before.

Nicotine, today found not only in cigarettes but also increasingly in vaping, is another. It stimulates our dopamine release, which in turn stimulates our reward centres, elevating our mood and our ability to think. The downside is that it is as addictive as cocaine and heroin and it reinforces the addiction by inducing craving. It also raises the pulse rate and blood pressure, thereby indirectly increasing the stress response rather than relieving it. Vaping has become popular on the grounds that it avoids all the cancer-causing effects of tobacco, yet vapers inhale far higher levels of nicotine than if they smoked cigarettes.

What most people do not know is that both caffeine and nicotine actually increase pain levels in pain sufferers. By ramping up our stress response, they sensitise the brain to pain and lower the threshold at which it is experienced. So, the very thing people think is helping to relieve their stress and pain is in fact reinforcing it.

Sugar is another stress reliever we turn to as, again, it gratifies our dopamine needs. Many coffee shops exploit this by selling you the coffee and the muffin, as well as the double shot of caramel syrup, sweetened cream and sprinkles. However, sugar also has its obvious drawbacks. Increased consumption of sugar and carbohydrates has led to an exponential rise in obesity. And, as we saw in the previous chapter, through a combination of hormonal responses and inflammation, obesity leads to painful joints and backache. In the case of knee pain, there is a direct relationship between kilos lost and a percentage reduction in pain felt, due not only to easing the load on the joint but also the decrease in circulating inflammatory cells, produced by the fat itself, which cause pain.

So, you can see that, even without being addicted to anything illegal, most of us spend our lives unwittingly boosting our dopamine levels, bouncing between caffeine, sugar and nicotine hits.

While discussing dopamine, we must also look at social media and the internet and their effects on us. It is well known that psychologists are employed in the digital industry to come up with ploys and strategies to attract us to whatever app, game or product they want us to buy. Knowledge is money in these cyber times and we 'netizens' are only too willing to hand over our data in return for some form of gratification. All too often that gratification is not in monetary form but a service that makes our life simpler or links us to things that we feel we need. In return, the tech providers use the data they glean from us to learn about how we behave or might respond if directed and pushed.

Facebook and Instagram know that every time someone gets a 'like' on their post, they get a dopamine surge which is equivalent to smoking two cigarettes. That's a reward for our efforts, and we want more of it. This 'want' and 'get' cycle gives rise to what is now called FOMO, fear of missing out. You scroll and scroll through the Instagram feed as it promises to deliver but so rarely does. However, the occasional reward is worth the hunt. We peer into the lives of others as if watching them on a highlights show-reel. Keeping up with friends, fren-emies and foes, we are convinced that everyone has a better life than we do, that they are all more successful and happier than we are. Younger generations have been led to believe that they have a right to be happy and if everyone else looks happier than they are, they feel a sense of loss and injustice. Which only reinforces their feelings of inadequacy, and makes them absorb more stress. The result is a need for more dopamine and so they look at their media and news feeds, while drinking their sugary drink, and the low mood and emotions which result stress them and ramp up their physical and mental pain.

Professor Jean Twenge conducted numerous studies over a period of 40 years, involving eight million teenagers.[55] Tracking each cohort between 1976 and 2016, she showed that since the introduction of smartphones teenagers are increasingly suffering behaviourally and emotionally from the effects of them. One study, which tracked their heart rate and breathing rate, showed that both of these increased significantly when they opened their social media. This was due to several factors but mostly to the sense of external obligation it induced, and the dopamine surges and falls brought about by notifications and messages. The term 'email or text apnoea' has been used to describe the breath-holding that occurs in anticipation of opening a message. Some of the symptoms experienced by social media addicts have been likened to those of mild PTSD. Instead of traumatic events, they are exposed to a stressful, 'always-on', interactive environment. They become unable to adjust to a more low-key and predictable life. Being plugged into constantly updated real time means always being primed to react. A study of smartphone 'withdrawal' discovered that people can become fidgety and anxious without their phones, and become over-sensitised to minor stimuli.

Clever marketing people have learned that most of us make decisions on the basis of what we 'feel', through our limbic centre (our mood and emotional centre), rather than what we 'think', using our logical, cognitive forebrains. As the well-known business speaker Simon Sinek says in his TED talk,[56] we are more interested in the 'why' of something than the 'what' or' how'. We quickly forget what people have said but we remember how they made us feel. However, emotional decision-making is, unfortunately, very unreliable as it is enormously open to bias. Behavioural psychologist Daniel Kahneman tells us that these decisions are based on heuristic (rule-of-thumb) tendencies and are unreliable and easily manipulated.[57]

In other words, whether we accept it or not we are being hacked. Yes, not only our computers but our brains, too. Companies like Google constantly watch our searching and buying behaviour and show us more of the type of thing we looked at before, to which they attach advertisements sensitive to our needs and wants. More importantly, they will never show us a countervailing argument or fact. So, what was a small bias or attitude in us becomes magnified the more we search. Brexit was an excellent example.

Even if you thought you were 'on the fence' regarding the debate and searched the pros of one option or the other, Google would polarise you to that argument. We unwittingly became a member of a 'tribe', entrenched in a set of beliefs on an emotional subject, to the point that, if later we find out we are wrong, we refuse to betray our fellows.

Once people have joined a group of this type, it is almost impossible to change their minds even if you show them the truth. And the reason that matters when we are talking about pain is because fixed thinking makes us more stressed by the points of view of others that contradict ours – basically, it makes us become more intransigent and entrenched in our views, and then, when we are crossed, we can't cope, so we become wary and don't know what to trust.

This was exemplified by the MMR (measles, mumps and rubella) vaccine controversy. You may remember that the discredited views of a British gastroenterologist, Dr Andrew Wakefield, led to a nationwide panic over the possibility that the combined vaccine could cause autism. This was later categorically disproved. And yet a recent study found that when parents who had not given their child the vaccine were shown unequivocal evidence that it was safe, and even admitted that their decision had been wrong, they still did not go on to get it done. They either found other negative reasons not to do it or refused because they somehow couldn't trust that the vaccine was OK.

I was contacted recently by a friend and colleague who is a GP. She was aware I was writing this book and we had discussed this topic of our being digitally hacked. She wanted me to know that she had realised that the online supermarket she used had known somehow that she was pregnant before she did.

How did that happen?

She explained that she had been surprised to find out that she was four months pregnant and had not realised because, although she had missed her periods, they had been very intermittent anyway. She had put her weight gain down to lack of exercise and a heavy workload. As she was so busy, she did her weekly shop online and had begun to notice that the advertisements flashing up on her screen were all for baby products: nappies, wet wipes, etc. She could not understand why, until she looked back through her orders for the previous few months and noticed that she had unwittingly been buying more carbohydrate-based and plainer foods, and not much that was spicy. The online shop's algorithm had spotted this change in her buying pattern and correlated it with women who are pregnant: hence the baby ads.

We are being more and more commercially and politically manipulated. And the ceaseless stream of news and facts, all of which promote a response in us, leads us to question what is true. The ability to get to the truth seems harder and harder; avoiding 'fake news' seems almost impossible – all of which contributes to our sense of disempowerment and loss of control over our lives and futures.

In the BBC documentary *HyperNormalisation*,[58] Adam Curtis takes us through an amazing visual, historical account of how the West has got to where it is today and how we feel in society. Curtis shows powerfully how we live in a time of great uncertainty and confusion. Events keep happening around us that seem inexplicable and out of control. The unexpected rise of Donald Trump, Brexit, the war in Syria, the endless migrant crisis, random bomb attacks... Those who are in power appear paralysed and have no idea what to do. We have retreated into a simplified and often completely fake version of the world; and, because it is all around us, we accept it as normal. Our perception is that finding the momentum to change is too unachievable, so we do nothing.

This sense of disempowerment and disenfranchisement is, along with social isolation, an important factor in the development of chronic pain. The Western, post-industrialised world has experienced peace for decades and no longer fears any real mortal danger. We are healthier and live longer than ever before, yet we and our children have become more emotionally vulnerable and sensitive and are no longer drawn together by shared hardship. We find it difficult to contextualise our experiences, which have become almost all emotional rather than physical. But as nature dictated, we are still competitive and have found ways of being so through our societal interactions.

This is not just through the portal of social media but also in how we lead our lives and educate our children. Recently, I was asked to attend an academic meeting with one of the tutors at my children's secondary school. It was designed to hear our views on how the school was run and what we thought was important in education. After reflection, I explained that what had struck me over the previous few years was how little of the work, particularly revision, ever seemed to be collaborative. Many of the students would have free study periods in which they worked in an isolated fashion. Such was the competition between them, often encouraged by the parents and the school, that they were terrified to admit to having any gaps or weaknesses in their knowledge. Rather than benefiting from helping each other outside the classroom, they withdrew into a world of their own to worry about what they did not know. It was as if, rather than working towards a common goal of achieving good grades in their A levels, they were striving towards a single award that only one person could win.

The same could be seen in their attitude to sport. Instead of working in cohesive groups, to achieve the best for the team, they were busy competing with each other, fearing failure, obsessed with making the grade for the 'A' team. The competition produces exactly the opposite effect required. The fear of failure produces risk aversion. They will not experiment to improve, and therefore they sabotage their own progress. Schools claim that they 'encourage their students to embrace failure', but very few actually create the culture or environment in which they can. This level of passive stress sensitises them and makes them tense, and later on their reluctance to show vulnerability spills over into their adult lives and heightens anxiety, and they turn up in clinics like mine with headaches and neck pain, like Max in the previous chapter. Pain in this instance arises from a need for protection from a subconscious sense of threat, but they cannot find safety, and so the pain persists.

There is gathering evidence in the fields of sociology and psychology that our ability to handle emotional responses starts early in childhood. This places even more pressure on parents to get it right within the limits of their busy schedules and the need to manage work and family life.

The areas of the brain responsible for the experience and

shaping of emotions develop in a child in response to parental involvement. The limbic system (our mood, emotional and sexual centre) matures by 'reading' and incorporating the emotional messages from the parent. Memory centres, both conscious and unconscious, rely on interaction with the parent for consolidation and for future interpretations of the world.

The templates for our future relationships are thus laid down by the relationships we have had with our earliest caregivers. The levels of sensitivity at which our pain systems are set consequently develop early, as our need for a protective alarm system is dependent on how protected we felt early in our development.

As Dr Gabor Maté says: 'We will understand ourselves as we have felt understood, love ourselves as we perceived being loved on the deepest unconscious levels, care for ourselves with as much compassion as, at our core, we perceived as young children.' [59]

In our hyper-stressed society, a child may feel that they do not have their parent's attention, even if the parent is sitting right next to them. This phenomenon, when the parent is physically present but emotionally absent, is known as proximate separation,[60] and is increasingly the norm. A good example, which I have witnessed many times, is the way parents behave on the school pick-up. This car time should be a very good opportunity for interaction and chatting but instead they are on their hands-free phones. Similarly, you see parents walking along the street, talking on their mobile phones with the child trailing behind. The level of stress imparted to the child through this phenomenon is believed to be as high as if the parent were physically separated from them. And, while this type of separation will not be recalled later in adult years or when looking back on childhood experience, it is nevertheless deeply etched as a sense of loss and often anger.

Neuroscientific studies using fMRI have shown that if we do not develop the ability to process emotions in our early years, we can be desensitised to future experiences. We now know that parts of the brain related to emotional behaviour are involved in pain states and that they are identically involved when submitted to stimuli that replicate the emotional conditions of pain but which do not involve any physical harm. The same areas of the brain also light up when physical harm occurs. That is to say, social and physical pain produce similar brain responses.

Such an effect was shown by neuroscientist Naomi Eisenberger, who tested the effect of social exclusion among a peer group.[61] While in a scanner, the subjects played a game of 'cyberball' in which they passed the ball to each other. Eisenberger was able to show that being excluded from the game caused brain activity similar to that which we would expect to see if the subjects were in physical pain.

The meaning-making processes that encompass the experience of physical pain appear to be the same as when we are experiencing such things as exclusion, bullying and grief. Social-emotional interactions greatly influence the development of the human brain. From birth they dictate the development and activity of the PNI system and, if poor, set up the potential for pain and illness in later years.

Parental touch and love are vital to their development. Young humans rely on adults much longer than the offspring of any other species, and not just as providers of food and shelter. They are also the biological regulators of the child's immature physiological and emotional systems. Parental love is not simply a warm and cosy experience; it is a biological necessity, essential for healthy physiological and psychological development. It ultimately drives the maturation of the circuitry of the brain.

Nature's aim is for the child to emerge as a self-sustaining, self-regulated human being who can live in harmony with fellow humans in a social context. Vital to this development is the relationship with the parent. Ultimately it will define how the adult child can cope with the stresses of their environment and the responses they mount to meet them, as well as the levels of fear they feel and the resultant pain they experience.

CASE HISTORY: ENZO

Enzo was a 28-year-old half-Italian man, who was fit and well. He still lived at home but had had some success in developing a niche dating app. He and his brother had a close relationship with their mother, who was divorced from their father.

Enzo was walking home one night and, as he looked one way to check for oncoming traffic in a small residential road, he was hit from the other side by a car which mounted the kerb and knocked his legs from under him. The driver did not stop. Enzo sustained a nasty fracture to his left knee and lower leg bone and tore all his major knee ligaments. His ankle was also fractured and dislocated. Enzo remembers nothing of the accident except waking to find the police standing over him and the wave of nauseating pain from his leg, which lay distorted, with his foot facing the wrong way – a sight he will never forget.

Until very recently, Enzo had been disturbed by repeated flashbacks of that night but had no memory of being hit or any details of the car or driver. In his dreams He described, in his dreams, the overpowering frustration of craning to try and see the car.

Enzo became obsessed with making as quick a recovery as possible and saw me weekly so I could put him through painful manipulation of his now healed but immobile knee and ankle. After three months of being in plaster, his leg was withered and wasted and he feared that he would never walk normally again.

We are putting the finishing touches on his last few degrees of movement, but I'm very proud of the work we have done with Enzo. He was recently reviewed at the hospital and found to be at least nine weeks ahead of his expected recovery. He is still racked by his lack of sleep and the constant need to repeat and relive the accident in his mind, which is producing erratic and aggressive behaviour. He's realised that having no memory of the accident deprived him of any means of coming to terms with how and why it happened. He feels he cannot leave behind the status of 'victim'. I referred him to an excellent psychologist who is an expert in PTSD and he is beginning to make good progress. We have tried to make Enzo see that the control and focus he has over his rehabilitation and the enormous success he has had with it is the control that he needs. It seems to be working. He needs to move forward with recovery rather than repeating the past.

CHAPTER 6

JACOB'S LADDER

(OR WHY BACK PAIN IS RARELY WHAT IT SEEMS)

'If your back was on your face you'd look after it.'
– Anon.

I have agonised over how to deal with this contentious sub-ject, partly because it is my particular interest – it is what I have specialised in in my clinical practice – but mainly because it just afflicts so many people. Of the 40 to 50 per cent of the population who suffer with chronic pain, 50 per cent report that it is in their spine.[62] The good news is that back pain is much more treatable in all its forms than people think. Even so, it represents a major burden on the state and the health system – not least because it comes in several forms, each requiring its own bespoke recipe of management. There is no single answer for all. Every back problem is unique, because we are.

As I sit here typing, I am mindful of the three lumbar

discs in my low back and the three cervical ones in my neck that are currently bulging and have been for several years. Two are pretty worn, to the extent that they have lost 75 per cent of their height and resemble a couple of old radial tyres, like those on the rather tired-looking bike sitting deflated and unused in my garage. I know this because I have been through all the usual rounds of MRI and CT scans, which have shown me sliced and diced in multiple dimensions, like the visual version of a salami machine, and given me amazing insight into the structure and condition of my spine. In fact, I have uploaded some of the images to the computer in my practice, to share with patients, not in a macabre way, but to reassure them that my spine is as bad, if not worse, in imaging terms, than theirs. I have to some extent 'been there'. In some way, this seems to validate me in their eyes as being experientially as well as professionally qualified to help them.

I do this because I do not want them to become victims of a phenomenon one of my colleagues calls 'V.O.M.I.T. syndrome' – Victim of Medical Imaging Technology. This is when patients become so absorbed and affected by what they have been shown on an X-ray or scan that they cannot disconnect from it visually. They begin to behave and live within the confines of what they *think* it means, rather than what it actually does mean. In my experience, patients are very visually impressionable and when they see the isolated image of a bulging or flattened degenerative disc, it becomes indelibly etched on their minds, particularly if an eminent specialist with letters after his name has reinforced the relevance of the 'injury' in worrying terms. Believe it or not, patients tend to feel more worried than reassured if we decide to use imaging. 'Blimey, he wants to MRI me… there must be something serious going on' tends to be the sentiment.

So, why do I have all of this imaging of myself? Well, as I wrote in the introduction to this book, I sustained a compression fracture to one of the vertebrae in my low back while playing rugby in my youth. I only discovered this when – the pain having become too much and with a growing weakness in the muscles of my left leg – I finally saw a spinal consultant, who sent me for imaging.

'Poor chap,' I hear you say. 'What agony he must be in!'

Thankfully, but not actually miraculously, I am not. In fact, most of the time I have no pain at all (and I have not needed imaging since). Apart from some occasional stiffness in my muscles, consistent with my life and sporting activities, as well as my age, my life is remarkably pain-free. Basically, I eat well, keep fit and slim, and more importantly, keep my back very strong and flexible. I accept that, like showering, shaving and cleaning my teeth in the morning, it is something I have to do to remain pain-free. I also know and accept that if I am going through a stressful period or sleeping poorly, or both, some of the old aches in my neck and back come home to roost for a while. They have become old friends that tell me all is not well in my world. I know that medication will not help because the pain is old and learned (chronic) rather than due to some new ache or injury.

And then very occasionally I have acute episodes, when my back goes into a rather deformed twist and I am limited in my daily activities, but it settles with time and I use all my little tricks of the trade to hasten its recovery. Each time it has been when I have let my maintenance routine slip for a month or two, mainly due to managing a busy clinical practice, which is very physical and emotional, as well as all my family activities and the stresses that life throws at me.

○ ○ ○

The human spine is an awesome and miraculous thing. It really is. It offers protection to the spinal cord and brain stem, while providing apertures for the nerves to pass into and out of the body, and multiple points of attachment for the myriad muscles that exert forces on it and enable us to stand erect. It allows multiple ranges of movement and provides the biomechanical base for our limbs to work from: our legs to walk and run; our arms and hands to feed us and operate devices requiring extreme dexterity and accuracy of motion and grip. It is capable of growing, adapting and changing on a daily basis even when you are older, not only in its fine structure but also in its density and strength. To give you some idea of the forces it is capable of withstanding, I have had patients who have undergone scoliosis surgery (to correct extreme developmental curves in the spine) – which involves inserting long titanium alloy rods along the spinal column, attached by screws – and who actually *break* the rods doing normal daily activities, while the bone those rods are there to support is unharmed. Living bone is strong, malleable and adaptable; 'plastic' is the term scientists use.

One myth we need to clear up is that the spine holds us up like a pylon supporting a bridge. It doesn't; it is much cleverer than that. The spine consists of 33 blocks of bone

– the vertebrae – held together in an 'S' bend front to back. It is not straight, and in fact, a flat, straight back can have as many problems as a too-curved one. These blocks are held together by a network of tough ligaments that tension it, while also allowing it to move in many directions. The muscles acting on it control the direction and degree of that movement, creating a supporting tension themselves at the same time.

We have two muscle systems: the ones that perform gross movements such as the biceps, which bend your arm at the elbow; and the deeper, more subtle system that fights our greatest enemy as *Homo sapiens*: gravity. This postural system does not – and cannot – fatigue; otherwise we would fall over. It has the ability to share 'shifts' of activity deep within the muscle, so that some fibres switch on while others rest and recover. It can, however, become weak if we sit or are inert for too long in our sedentary working lives and, as it struggles to keep up, we experience this breakdown as a dull ache.

Between the bony blocks are the discs. They are mainly made of cartilage and, amazingly, consist of 60 per cent water. Overnight the discs recover somewhat and imbibe fluid from their environment. They thus slightly reinflate during sleeping hours and so we are technically taller in the morning than in the evening. The cartilage, the *annulus fibrosus* (a bit like the silicone sealant you use in bathrooms in consistency), is laid down in concentric rings in different directions, much like the radial tyre I described earlier; while the centre of the disc (the *nucleus pulposus*) is made of a pulpy substance with a consistency similar to toothpaste. In fact, the discs behave at times much like a car tyre, and at others like a chocolate with a soft centre, as you'll see if you read on…

When a load is applied to the discs, they compress a little, much like a tyre. The rings absorb the load and the soft centre exerts pressure outwards as the cartilage exerts it inwards. There is an equilibrium in pressure and the disc is very strong and stable. But actually most of the bodily pressure is taken up by our core muscles, which provide a corset of cylindrical stability through the abdomen, diaphragm and spinal muscles: in a perfect, athletic spine, very little pressure should be put through the discs. The rest of the large movements of the spine, such as bending, twisting and lifting, are performed by chains of muscles linked all the way from the legs and low back to the upper torso. One of these, the posterior chain, consists basically of the core abdominal muscles, hamstrings, gluteal muscles, deep low back and loin muscles, as well as the laterals, traps and neck muscles.

Each muscular group making up these chains is linked by fascinating stuff called fascia. I guess that makes it 'fascia-nating' (sorry!) This can be likened to tough cling-film, except that it is thick and ungiving. It permeates through the muscle chains and links them to provide tension. It is the membrane stuff you peel off a chicken breast before cooking it.

This whole complex structure works through a system we call *tensegrity* – integrity through tension. The concept is used in modern engineering for bridges and cranes but nature invented it long before we did.

To get an idea of how it works, look at the image opposite of the child's toy called a Jacob's ladder (Figure

5). It consists of a series of wooden tiles joined together by ribbons which weave between them in a snake pattern. The tiles are not glued or stuck in any way but held within the ribbons by tension alone. If you invert one of the tiles it tumbles down the chain but is still held within the ribbons by the tension on them. Magic!

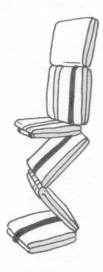

Figure 5: Jacob's Ladder

So, we have to look at the spine as an integrated functional system of support, protection and locomotion. It is self-nourishing and repairing and has all the tools it needs to adapt and heal itself. Evolution has seen to it that there is very little in our bodies that is superfluous to requirements and, indeed, many of the body's structures fulfil supplementary functions. For example, the diaphragm, the dome-shaped muscle whose primary purpose is to allow us to breathe, has a secondary function of compressing and pumping the stomach and bowel, assisting the mechanical breakdown of food, and aiding the passage of food along the bowel, by pressing down on the stomach wall beneath it. This is borne out in the necessity to strain and hold one's breath while passing a stool. But let's not get too graphic. The diaphragm is partly attached to the spine and if it gets very tight from poor breathing it will manifest in locking the spine at that level and causing pain.

This type of dysfunction is what osteopaths, like me, treat all day long. Philosophically, we do not divorce the musculoskeletal system from any other system.

BACK AND DISC INJURIES (USUALLY ACUTE)

Let's get trauma out of the way. I have one rule that I teach my students about trauma to the brain, spine, or indeed any bone. If someone reports immediate pain that continues at the same level after a fall or a blow, particularly at night, then it is a fracture until proven otherwise and needs to be imaged, at least X-rayed. This is particularly the case in the elderly and the very young. Old people are brittle and young bones have growth plates and are apt to hide injury within their flexibility. This rule has never let me down and I am only too happy to be wrong.

Obviously, trauma is a particular situation. What I want to look at here is what happens to the vertebral discs, first as a natural process, and then when they get injured.

Imagine placing a strawberry-cream-filled chocolate between your thumb and index finger and gently squeezing it so that it slightly flattens but stays intact: that is what happens to a disc when it is loaded or as we get older. The chocolate sides will bulge very slightly. This effect occurs slowly and over time and there is nothing about it that causes acute disturbance of its structure or any neighbouring structure and therefore no inflammatory response is needed. As a result, neither of these events cause pain… ever! So, although they account for about 90 per cent of the bulges you will see in spines on MRI scans, and are often cited as the cause of pain, they are nothing to worry about.

Likewise, as part of a natural and *normal* process, partly genetic and partly due to time and how much you abuse your back, discs lose their water content and thus become drier. This process can produce micro-cracks within them, again very like an old rubber tyre. Pressure on these cracks creates the potential for bulges to form. This does not matter at the front of the disc as there are no nerves to be irritated. At the back of the disc, the biggest cause of bulges is sitting, because of the uneven pressure put on it, which encourages it to push backwards over time. But even when the discs do bulge significantly, so that they nudge a nerve, if this happens slowly, the nerve can move over and assume a better position. And, unless the patient complains of pain consistent with the distribution of that nerve, it is irrelevant.

I saw a great example of this in a Formula One driver a few years ago while I was working as a human performance advisor to the team. We performed baseline scanning of the drivers' spines to spot potential problems that might be a risk to them when their bodies were placed under the extreme G-forces of racing. We were gobsmacked to find that one driver had such an enormous disc prolapse in his low back that the path of the nerve was almost indiscernible. Yet he had never complained of any pain in his back or leg. The only reason for this that we could come up with was that the disc, though bulging and distorted, had not actually ruptured, so no inflammatory response had been mounted. Though the nerve was compressed to half its width, it could still move within the hole it exited through, so it was happy. Also, the driver was supremely fit with a very strong core and back.

To ram this home, I want to give you a stat. In 2014, researchers at the famous Mayo Clinic in the US found that disc degeneration was normal at *all* ages.[63] 'Black' (which is how they look on MRI scans), dehydrated discs were present in a third of 20-year-olds who had no symptoms at all. It was there in 96 per cent of 80-year-olds, also with no back pain. The Mayo concluded that these findings were not 'part of a pathological process requiring intervention' – medical-speak for, 'if you see them do nothing'.

○ ○ ○

Back to the chocolate cream. Keep squeezing it until a small crack appears in the bulge but the centre does not actually leak out. That is what we call in the trade a disc (annular) tear with a small herniation (protrusion). These tears can occur suddenly after repetitive straining or lifting (gardening, sweeping), and are often painful, but rarely compress nerves, so the pain stays in the back and does not travel down a leg. This sudden disruption causes inflammation and produces chemicals that irritate the outer layer of the spinal cord and a small network of fine nerves that supply the back of the disc. The tears are visible on a scan, appearing as a 'lit up' section within the bulge and telling us that the injury is new and inflamed. There is usually accompanying spasm and a lot of pain, with a barrage of 'worry' messages being sent to the brain (nociception). Unfortunately, spinal discs have a very bad blood supply, which means that the tears take longer to heal than in other soft tissues, but they do heal. A bad muscle tear, for example, will take three weeks to heal because it has a rich supply of blood vessels to activate and supply healing cells and nutrients. The average disc tear will take eight to twelve weeks to settle, though, if well managed, most people will see a big improvement after three weeks.

Do they need an MRI?... Nope. Any back specialist worth their salt can work out the nature of the injury from a good case history and clinical examination. As for the treatment, rehabilitation and strengthening of the back and core is vital. But complete immobilisation (bed rest) is a disaster – keeping moving as much as possible is best. We also need to educate the patient not to fear the pain or its recurrence. I am a big fan of helping patients with pain relief in the form of painkillers and anti-inflammatories as it allows them to feel better while nature takes its course. There is evidence that anti-inflammatories slow healing, but in my experience not by much, and the patient is happy to forgo a few days of healing if they are in much less pain. I also think that any delay in healing is offset by their ability to keep moving and initiate special exercises. Even more importantly, the quicker you stall or prevent too much nociception (receptors firing into the cord and brain) entering the nervous system, the less likely that this will get established centrally in the brain and become chronic or persistent pain later.

Many patients will respond well to over-the-counter medicines such as ibuprofen but often use them wrongly by taking them only when the pain is bad instead of keeping a constant preventive level of it their bloodstream, which is more effective. Imagine that the tiny dose has to get all the way through your gut and around the body to get to the target tissue and do its thing.

Good manual therapy is also very useful after the first week, but not before. However, chiropractic-style 'cracking' at this stage is a no-no and may make it worse. Ultrasound and laser therapy are a complete waste of time for back pain; any perceived improvement is placebo. Of course, some would argue that if the placebo effect results in relief to the patient, why not do it? We will come to that in Chapter 9.

Now, if you overdo it and squeeze the chocolate too hard, the strawberry cream will spill out through the crack in the chocolate. Likewise, when a tear appears in the disc wall, the contents can potentially leak on to and compress the nerves on either side of it, which are very susceptible to irritation and are pain-sensitive. These nerves supply power and sensation to the muscles in the leg. Eighty per cent of these tear injuries occur in one of the two last discs in the low back. The most common symptom is pain in the back of one leg, known as sciatica, though this is a general term.

In most cases, the sciatica too will ease as the immediate

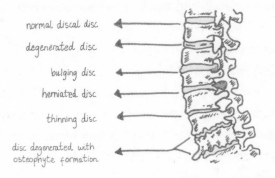

Figure 6. Stages of degeneration of a disc from top to bottom. Believe it or not, most of these will not cause pain if the back and core are kept strong.

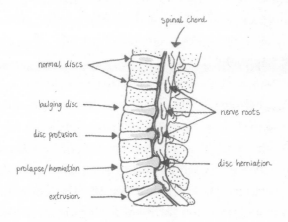

Figure 7. Different degrees of disc bulging. Again, all may be pain-free.

inflammation and swelling in the disc settles and the compression retracts. However, this type of nerve pain can be horrendous and really gets to you. And, in my experience, this is when patients are most vulnerable and susceptible to giving into surgery. If their pain is not managed, they will agree to almost anything to get rid of it, only to regret it later. Psychological mood and resilience are very low and sleep is poor. I know; I have been there.

If the compression is severe, it interferes with the transmission of impulses in the nerve and will affect sensory perception and be felt as pins and needles or numbness in the distribution of that nerve. In rare cases, the motor fibres to the muscles are affected, with resultant weakness in them. Footdrop, which results in the inability to lift the foot off the ground, is an example of this. It is extremely debilitating and disabling and it is often necessary to operate to remove the disc, as the nerve can be permanently damaged if not relieved quickly.

There is only one other acute necessity for surgery and that is when the disc has effectively herniated so much that it occupies a large section of the canal space which should house the base of the spinal cord. We call it the *cauda equina* (horse's tail) because at this level there is no actual spinal cord, only a skein-like bundle of nerve roots. Again, this is very rare but does happen and can cause loss of urinary and bowel function, as well as loss of sensation to the nether regions and erectile dysfunction. Such symptoms require urgent assessment with an MRI scan and a neurosurgeon. Cauda equina syndrome usually happens because the nerves are compressed acutely and without warning. I say this because it is quite common to find, almost incidentally, that patients have compression of the same nerves by slow bony overgrowth into the canal (*canal stenosis*) equivalent to that of the acute disc. However, they have no symptoms at all. This is because in this case, with time, the nerve roots can adopt a new position and adapt to the squeeze. Here, the scan should be used to confirm the diagnosis only if symptoms develop and based on a good clinical examination.

The other anatomical structure in the spine most commonly involved in back pain is the facet joint (Figure 8 below). Each vertebra is linked by two sets of facet joints. One pair faces upward and one downward. They are located at the back of the spine, and have a flat face, lined with cartilage. They are synovial joints, which means that they can get inflamed and cause pain as they have a membrane around them (the capsule) which is pain-sensitive. This capsule is supplied by a hair-like nerve called the medial branch.

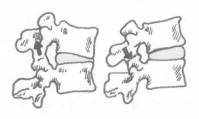

Figure 8. The arrows indicate the facet joints opening
and closing with movement.

These joints are easily irritated by repetitive loaded movements, particularly if they are one-sided or asymmetrical or involve rotation, such as in golf and tennis.

In the neck, they can become painful from poor posture, working at laptops, overuse of smartphones or sleeping on your front. Over time, they can become arthritic and produce bony spurs, which resemble the edge of an oyster shell. And, if not supported by good surrounding muscles, the joints can become irritated and painful. However, as with discs, on scans we regularly see degenerative joints that are not causing any pain. For me in clinic, the biggest giveaway of facet joint-mediated pain is the associated wasting of the deep spinal muscle also visible on the scan. This usually indicates that a reflex has developed between the pain and the spinal cord that has shut down those muscles as a protective response. Treatment must be aimed at not only settling the irritation of the joints but also 'waking up' and dramatically increasing the strength of the affected muscles. Only this will give prolonged relief and prevent recurrence.

The spine needs to be stable in many ranges of movement, including bending and twisting, but equally this is when most injuries occur. This is because most of our daily activities, including a lot of the exercise we do, involve only one plane of movement. The three sports that most commonly set off backs are golf, tennis and football; all of them involve multiple rotation and side-bending, which we do not do all week. Then at the weekend we are surprised when something goes twang when we perform aggressive movements that our backs are not ready for. Often the pain emanates not from a structural injury, but from the brain telling us that our tissues are becoming strained and will potentially get injured. The pain is protective rather than an emergency.

The important thing to take away here is that almost all back pain is avoidable. Being flexible and strong as well as slim and active is vital. Realising that many of the things that you do at work or play involve 'habit', in terms of how you use your muscles, is key. Even if you cannot change an action you have to perform, do stretches to prevent muscles you overuse from tightening. Even sitting on a sofa which is offset to the TV will produce neck or low back pain if you constantly have to rotate to face the screen. Similarly, jobs such as working as a cashier in a supermarket or bank often involve reaching and turning while your chair is facing in a fixed direction. Asymmetries in muscle tension can develop and produce pain. So, move either yourself or the screen and stretch as much as possible.

The real problem is that most of us are lazy. I know that sounds harsh but it's true. Hand on heart, most of us know we do not look after ourselves. We wait for something to happen and react rather than being proactive. Anyone in the world of physical medicine will tell you that getting patients to do what you tell them is the most difficult thing to achieve. Yet they are very quick to complain when it all goes wrong! You have to see yourself as a finely tuned sports car. You can either go on to become an equally tuned vintage car, admired and coveted by all, or end up a rusty old jalopy destined for the crushers. It's all about maintenance: with just a bit of servicing and a regular polish, the engine will keep firing and work well for its years. You can moan at the boss about desks and ergonomics, but you are driving the car and responsible for it.

At the other extreme, we have the Iron Man-loving, ultramarathon loonies, who shake their joints to bits and push their physiology to the limits for too long. It becomes an obsession that takes over their lives. They come to the clinic and say: 'It only hurts when I run 20 kilometres, Doc.' Deep down inside I want to respond: 'Well, run five and bog off.' I can only say this because I have been there too. Some years back, I trained fanatically and got to the point where I felt constantly tired, with muscle and joint fatigue, and was too busy training to see my wife and family and ended up with a heart arrhythmia, which I had to have fixed. So, one day, at the end of an ultramarathon, with my body screaming at me, I did a Forrest Gump and just stopped. I looked up at the sky, asked myself who I was proving myself to and whether I was going to wait for my knees to give out before I realised my madness. I threw my trainers in the bin by the finishing line and began to enjoy life once more.

Moderation, as my grandmother always said, is the key to everything.

So, as far as acute pain is concerned, it *should* be easy to avoid, but do not worry unduly if it happens; in about 85 per cent of cases it will settle down with time and treatment. Very few back problems should ever need to be referred to a specialist, and often that can be a slippery slope to surgery. But do get professional advice from a therapist or doctor and choose someone who knows how to use their hands for manual therapy. And don't be afraid of short-term medication for pain, as it will help get you moving. Start with the chemist and go to the GP only if the low-level medication is not cutting it.

- If the practitioner wants to use imaging immediately, ask

why and what they are looking for. If they can't provide a reason of concern, they either don't know what's going on or they have some other incentive, in which case don't go back.

• If they don't examine you, or if they ask you to pay up front, don't go back.

• If they keep taking X-rays and talking about small alignment issues, don't go back. You won't get any better in the long term – and you will end up glowing in the dark!

• There is no such thing as a perfect spine on imaging. It's the functioning of it that matters.

• If a practitioner is defensive or impatient, they don't see therapy as a partnership and are not empowering you with knowledge and control. Don't go back.

• If they tell you: 'You are lucky not to be in a wheelchair,' don't go back.

• If you ask for a second opinion, they should welcome it. If they are correct in their diagnosis, then another professional should agree with them and reassure you that you are with the right person.

• Knowledge is everything and there are some great books out there, many of which are in 'Further Reading' at the back of this book.

• Most importantly, as Corporal Jones said in *Dad's Army,* 'Don't panic!' It never helps and mostly makes things worse. Pain rarely means serious harm. Breathe and get some help. Call on friends to help. Don't be a hermit; isolation only makes things worse and depresses you.

• Lastly, unless you are screaming like a banshee, don't take to your bed. If you absolutely have to, get up every half-hour.

PERSISTENT (CHRONIC) BACK PAIN

So now the biggy – chronic or, as I prefer to call it, persistent back pain. The one that just doesn't seem to get better. Incidentally, there is a whole vocabulary around pain and backs that is depressing in its very essence, and I would have an industry-wide change of terminology if I could. Words like 'chronic' and 'degenerative' should come with a health warning; for me, and most of my patients, they conjure up misery and the 'beginning of the end'. Radiology reports on X-rays and scans are particularly guilty of this. They use long, complicated and depressing terms to describe findings that are actually quite normal for the age and sex of the patient.

Jeffrey G Jarvik, a marvellously innovative neuro-radiologist in the US, once tried an experiment with his report writing. He included a message that read: 'The following findings are so common in people without low back pain that while we report their presence, they must be interpreted with caution and in the context of the clinical situation.' [64]

Jarvik was surprised to observe on follow-up that the patients whose reports contained his message were significantly less likely to pursue other medical investigations or to have repeated imaging. Furthermore, they were less likely to get follow-up prescriptions for strong medications. Extraordinarily, having understood that the pain did not reflect a dangerous pathological process, they felt confident enough to pursue exercise and other rehabilitative strategies.

One of the things I find astounding about the current chronic pain crisis is that much of the medical world is blissfully unaware of its prevalence. One reason for this is the '90/10 rule', a concept that arose from some research into people with back pain who went to see their doctors. The study found that 90 per cent of the millions of people seeing their doctor each year about back pain recovered on their own within two to three months. People with back pain get better...[65]

...Or maybe not. Further research in the UK by epidemiologist Peter Croft, director of Keele University's Primary Care Research Centre,[66] showed that this data was highly unreliable. In his estimation, only a quarter of back pain patients recovered within a year. It was true that 90 per cent of them did not return to their doctor within three months but this was not because they had resolved the problem. It was because they had simply given up on primary care as a source of help and moved on to other types of practitioner and interventions. This shows just how much conventional medicine has lost track of the problem.

Pretty much all persistent pain was once acute pain that was simply not treated quickly enough. Almost all of it manifests in soft tissues rather than bone. Most acute pain settles and disappears. However, for some – and it would appear to be a very significant number – that pain undergoes change, and something makes it persist. For us in the medical world working with pain, finding out who those people are, so that we can help prevent the crossing of the Styx into the underworld of suffering, is the key issue.

In many cases, the acute episode is just the straw that breaks the camel's back. And what really matters is the state that many of us get ourselves into as a backdrop to the episode. One of the major problems that society faces today is that 80 per cent of us sit all day and often for most of the evening, too. Sitting around for most of the day has become as deadly as smoking or obesity. *The Lancet* medical journal reported that too much sitting increased risk of mortality by 59 per cent. About 5 million deaths globally each year can be attributed to prolonged sitting. This is similar to the level found for obesity and smoking.[67]

Microbiologist Marc Hamilton at the University of Missouri-Columbia is a researcher into the effects of inactivity, and as he puts it, 'sitting too much is not the same as exercising too little.'[68] This is because when sitting the legs are inactive and we do not use the specialised leg muscles known as the 'deep red quadriceps', and there is rapid loss of a vital enzyme that helps remove fat and cholesterol from the bloodstream.

The general and wide-ranging effects of doing nothing are catastrophic in the long term. And in the shorter term, the stasis in our bodies caused by inactivity, as well as the wasting and deconditioning of the muscles in our legs, backs and abdomens, predisposes us to developing pain. How does this happen without us actually injuring ourselves? After all, sitting at a desk can't tear muscle or strain ligaments. Well, it's a set of different effects. When people sit, they place three times the pressure through the back of the spinal discs as when they stand and move. Sitting slumped is even worse. Over a prolonged period, bulges develop in the discs and the ligaments, which hold them in, slacken and stretch them. This in itself is not painful, but once the back of the disc is weakened, it is vulnerable to the larger movements we do when we are more active, perhaps playing sports or gardening at the weekend. Add into the pot the weakening of the stabilising system of the spine, the abdomen and back muscles, and it's a recipe for disaster. Disc injuries can occur acutely as a result, and these will settle, as we have discussed. But most people will be satisfied once the pain has gone and go on living their lives without ever changing how they look after their backs or establishing a regular exercise programme or stretching. And, as the saying goes, if you do what you always do, you will get what you always get. On the other hand, many also believe, quite wrongly, that if they do certain things it will all happen again and so they shut down their activity, thinking it is a protective strategy. The cycle of fear and protection begins.

There are additional effects beyond what happens specifically to the discs. Most of us, as we have discussed earlier, sit racing our engines and going nowhere. We often work under a lot of stress, physiologically producing all the adrenaline-filled normal responses of being chased by a mammoth but not actually acting on it physically. Our bowels shut down, our muscles tense across our entire bodies, without us being aware of it, and our 'thinking' brain centres shut down by about 25 to 30 per cent. Pain-firing trigger points pop up in our muscles and seem to spread, which makes us think something much more sinister is going on. Isolated back pain seems to creep to other areas. Over time, our immune systems are impaired, so we get more infection and colds, and inflammation increases, so that our joints and backs hurt more. The changes in our breathing patterns (hyperventilation and breath-holding) produce tension in our necks, which results in headaches and dizziness, and we clench our teeth at night, so that our jaws and craniums ache and we sleep poorly. Consequently, we don't get good recovery-type sleep. The glass of wine we take to help us drift off into the world of Morpheus only makes things worse, as it prevents the natural wave-like changes between deep and shallow sleep that we need, to rationalise all the day's events and store memory. Before we know it, we have gone into what I call the *Corti-zone.*

Once the stress hormone, cortisol, is pumping around us, we store fat in our abdomens. As we put on weight, the increased inflammation generated by the fat causes pain in the back and joints, as well as loading them with more to carry. It also causes cholesterol to line our blood vessels. We seek greater and greater gratification in the form of sugar and other carbohydrates, because we don't feel good. We may drink caffeine, smoke and vape more to get more dopamine and happy brain chemicals. The short-term effect is outweighed by the stimulants ramping up our pain. Basically, we go into a state of long-term physiological 'hypervigilance', which becomes a habit we can't shake off. We know it is happening as we look in the mirror and see bags around our eyes and pallid skin and wonder at the how the doughnut we had for elevenses has miraculously reformed as a ring around our bellies. For some of us, the lack of control over our lives and the realisation we may never get out of the rut we are in only heighten our anxiety and tension. Our emotionally based limbic and pain systems switch on and we sensitise further to the pain we already feel. Our emotion filter becomes more sensitive and our moods swing randomly. The pain seems to spread and intensify as our brains undergo central sensitisation (the top-down process we talked about in Chapter 1) and even in the periphery our neurones change the receptors on them so that they fire more for less and turn up the neuro-volume knob.

As a result of this, what was a background level of altered state is now escalated by the acute episode. The tsunami wave of pain swamps us and our 'cope-ability' is exhausted. We are left in a pain state that does not go away, even though the actual injury has long since healed. Welcome to the world of seemingly interminable back pain, fibromyalgia, IBS, migraine, fatigue and depression. They are all basically the same thing presenting in different ways.

But... before you descend into a black hole of despair and helplessness, if you read back over this chapter, you will realise that it is all changeable, manageable and curable. It's just about knowing that in order to heal ourselves we need to take steps to change many variables in our lives, not just our workstation. If you make that mindset adjustment and see that it is possible, then it will become entirely more probable. As Frank Vertosick says in his book *Why We Hurt*: 'We must try to shed the chains of pain, cloak our souls against the cold, and continue to climb our mountains.'[69]

CASE HISTORY: PAMELA

I first heard about Pamela from her niece, a patient of mine. Pamela was 80 years old and had been living alone since being widowed 20 years previously. She belonged to that war-time generation, raised on rationing and making-do, for whom independence was an absolute priority. She had never spent a night in hospital in her life. She lived in a bungalow and tended the quarter acre of land surrounding it without any assistance. She frequently did at least the recommended 10,000 steps a day walking her two dogs; and for journeys to the village a mile away, she rode a sit-up-and-beg bike, rather like Miss Marple. Also, like Miss Marple, she spurned wearing a cycle helmet.

The trouble began when a Pilates class started up in the village hall. Pamela went along and enjoyed it at first. But then a local group of yummy mummies joined and started demanding harder exercises. Pamela gamely carried on attending until, after a particularly tough class, she woke in the night with such pain in her low back, pelvis and right leg that she had to phone her son for help. Her GP told her it was her age and prescribed bed rest and strong painkillers, which made her feel anxious and woozy and brought on fears of dementia.

So, Pamela booked an appointment with a chiropractor in the next town. She was initially reassured when the practitioner didn't dismiss her fears: he took a full medical history and sent her for an X-ray. But when she went back, it was to alarming news. The chiropractor showed her the image of her spine, which Pamela could see was anything but the smooth, straight supportive structure she had in her mind. The chiropractor told her she had scoliosis, bone spurs and herniated discs, which were compressing nerves, and which would get worse if she did not act quickly. With a course of 12 treatments, he promised he would render her pain-free.

Pamela had always been very careful with her money but when she thought of what it would cost her to have someone to do her garden if she couldn't manage it, 12 treatments seemed like a bargain, so she paid upfront. Sure enough, after 10 sessions she did feel better – though she still got leg pain if she did too much – and she appreciated the interest the practitioner took in her life. But when the course of treatments came to an end, the chiropractor recommended another course as preventive treatment. Luckily, before paying up, Pamela happened to mention this to her niece, who mentioned it to me and asked if I would take a look at her aunt before she handed over any more money.

This I was happy to do. I examined her and took a full case history and established that, prior to the Pilates problem, Pamela had lived an active life that belied her years. So, unless she had randomly experienced a compression fracture or developed some rare disease, which her history told me she had not, the pain had a mechanical or soft-tissue origin. I didn't go over her X-ray, which she had with her, but said I would look at it later. I didn't want to reinforce her idea of having a 'crumbling spine', as she called it. However, I showed her my own low back X-ray, which, she had to agree, was worse than hers even though she had 30 years on me. Thorough examination confirmed that she had no signs of fracture or nerve compression; in fact, I could get her leg 90 degrees in the air.

Furthermore, she never complained of any pins and needles or numbness, which would correlate with nerve involvement. Hunting for trigger points, I found some scorchers in her hip muscles, which referred pain straight down her leg in the distribution she complained of. These were likely to have been activated by a particular exercise she had been given in Pilates, which had tightened up already overactive muscles.

Gentle treatment to release these trigger points gave her instant relief and I showed her how to work on them herself over the next ten days to further relieve them. I also gave her very specific exercises to wake up some lazy muscles in her hips and legs and to stabilise and strengthen her low back. I advised her to give up not only the chiropractor but also the Pilates for a while, as it had been too generic for her and she needed exercise to be more specific to her personal issues. The class had become too big for the instructor to monitor all the participants. Perhaps she could spend her money on a few one-to-one sessions after I had had a quick chat with the instructor to guide the rehab? We also put her in touch with a t'ai chi class in her area.

As a parting shot, I suggested that if she really wanted to live to be 100, then wearing a cycle helmet might be a good idea, too. Her niece tells me Pamela has taken up t'ai chi and has no pain, but the cycle helmet she bought her hangs unused on the coat peg.

CHAPTER 7

GHOSTS IN THE MACHINE

'Some of us have wounds that have never healed. We have
lived with them so long that we don't even know they are
there any more. But pain reminds us.'

– 'Tuck' in *The Best of Me*

After back pain, there is a whole host of other chronic
pain-related conditions that cause widespread misery, place
a strain on health services and have such a profound effect
on sufferers' lives that in some cases they are unable to hold
down a job or maintain a relationship. If you are a sufferer
of fibromyalgia, chronic fatigue syndrome (CFS), irritable
bowel syndrome (IBS) or migraine, then you have doubt-
less spent years, decades even, pursuing relief to no avail.
You have almost certainly become cynical about promises
of a cure – and enraged by those practitioners who tell you
'It's all in the mind.'

Don't worry: I'm not going to hold out false hope.
Nor am I going to promise you can think yourself better.
Instead, I hope to show you that underlying those symp-

toms as distinct as blinding headaches, painful joints or exhaustion, there are some uniting factors at work. And if we understand those, then relief is possible. I am also going to introduce you to hypermobility, which commonly intertwines with the roots of these chronic conditions.

As I said in Chapter 1, the current biomedical model of medicine is not comfortable around conditions that are not explained by a tangible, identifiable underlying disease, i.e. that do not fall within the realms of biology, surgery or pharmacology alone. As a result, medicine tends to mistrust the patient's story if it does not match the clinical findings. The patient gets filed under neurotic or 'malingerer'.

But, either way, stating baldly that 'there is currently no known cure', as the NHS website does for fibromyalgia, is depressing and completely self-defeating.[70] A more helpful approach would be: 'We have given a set of symptoms and a pain syndrome an official Latin name but don't know how to treat it within the confines of our knowledge because it falls into a grey area and we don't like grey areas.'

FIBROMYALGIA

First, let's take a look at fibromyalgia. If we accept that what I have presented so far in this book is the mode by which pain, fatigue and related depression can develop, then fibromyalgia is not difficult to understand. It is characterised by persistent widespread musculoskeletal pain, a phenomenon called allodynia (increased pain sensitivity), and trigger points in defined areas of the body, one of which must present with a score of 11 out of 18 to qualify for diagnosis. It affects significantly more women than men and sufferers often complain of insomnia, fatigue, anxiety, depression, gastrointestinal symptoms and headaches, as well as 'fibro-fog', an unpleasant loss of mental functioning and acuity that manifests as memory loss and slower recall of names and places.

At the heart of fibromyalgia lies the world of *central sensitisation*, which we covered in Chapter 2, but which I will recap and summarise for you again here. This is when the brain, through repeated failure to come to terms with whatever threat or lack of safety it perceives, gets trapped in a vicious cycle of arousal, the sources of which are due partly to childhood experiences and partly to current environmental circumstances (our lives, basically). As a result, three things happen physiologically:

1. The firing threshold of the nervous system lowers and smaller stimuli cause pain.

2. The after-effect of pain lingers; and episodes merge and become constant.

3. Previously harmless input from the tissues to the brain is interpreted as harmful or noxious.

CFS, IBS and migraine often co-exist with fibromyalgia, and they all have the same causation or origin. They are effectively all pain syndromes, and muscle is the common denominator in all three.

IBS OR 'GUT FEELINGS GONE MAD'

IBS or irritable bowel syndrome afflicts around 15 per cent of the industrialised world and it is the most common reason that patients are referred to gastroenterologists.[71]

It is a set of unpleasant and debilitating symptoms (not a disease) which can include abdominal cramps, bloating, diarrhoea, constipation, or both intermittently. Its associated symptoms are tiredness, nausea, heartburn and indigestion, needing to pass urine frequently, backache, muscle pains, headaches, anxiety and depression. Quite a mix, and that's the interesting bit. Because, although the primary symptoms manifest in the bowel, the syndrome overlaps into several other systems.

If we take 'backache', which we associate with coming from the tissues and muscles of the spine (the musculoskeletal system), this may seem unrelated, as a symptom, to the bowel. But it is not. The backache occurs through a reflex we call a 'visceral reflex'. The part of the bowel which becomes irritated refers the pain back through the nerve which supplies it, to the level of the spine (the low back area) from which the nerve takes its origin. This nerve becomes hyper-aroused and 'switches on' along its whole length – to such an extent or threshold that the brain registers pain in all of the regions the nerve supplies. In the same way, the pain of a menstrual period is often not only felt in the lower abdomen but also sets off backache.

Although a large proportion of IBS patients present to tummy specialists, many who have the condition are never seen by doctors, so figures for the prevalence of this condition are probably conservative to say the least. When fMRI brain scans are carried out on these patients,[72] it is common to find that an unusual part of the brain lights up in them when the abdominal pain is felt. This region is known as the prefrontal cortex and is associated with the storage of emotional memories. Therefore, we can reasonably conclude that some event of emotional importance is occurring because of, and at the same time as, the pain being felt, which is a result of the automatic firing of nerve pathways formed and sensitised long ago. How can we account for the formation of these pathways? There is a strong association in these cases of abusive or unhappy childhoods, as well as chronic stress in adult life.[73]

Just as fibromyalgia is characterised by global bodily muscular pain and sensitive trigger points in the muscles, the pain of IBS is stimulated by tension within the muscles of the bowel wall. As the bowel contracts (a movement known as peristalsis), pain is felt, and activation of the skeletal muscles hurts on movement. At the same time, because stress responses cause the vagus nerve (the principal nerve of our 'rest-and-digest' system) to shut down, bowel movements also shut down partially and become disordered in their rhythm. The receptors within them become sensitised and volatile. Digestion is interrupted and the bowel wall becomes *ischaemic*, which means it does not receive enough oxygen and so metabolic waste products build up. This is painful and can cause inflammation in the bowel wall. After a while, these changes also interfere with the absorption of nutrients from the food being digested, resulting in variable bowel movements, from constipation to diarrhoea.

We would be wrong, however, to think that IBS is a disease of muscle. Rather, it is due to the hyper-aroused state of the nervous system and the way it is communicating with the gut, through the pathways that I have described in previous chapters. Remember that the gut does a lot more than digest food. It is also an important sensory organ that we switch on when we are stressed in order to better assess threat from external environmental elements. In fact, there are more nerves running from the gut to the brain than from the brain to the gut – hence what we nonchalantly call 'gut feeling', which is actually a real and rather fascinating phenomenon.

Most of the time we recognise a gut feeling as a message that something is 'up'. That 'something' could range from an excited stirring of the loins to a revolted response at something we have just seen or even the harbinger of impending doom. Whichever emotion it represents, it is a warning to prepare, be ready or protect. As we have already discussed, the bowel, including the stomach, despite our perception that it is within us, is in fact a portal through which infections or toxins can invade from outside. It directly interacts with our environment. So the brain has, by necessity, to place a high level of vigilance around its entire length as a monitoring system for threat. Through a branch of the PNI system (see page 88) the brain and gut have a constant conversation.

It is if that stress response goes on for too long that changes occur in the gut and it remains in a 'fight or flight' status. Like any sensory organ, it can become sensitised and fire pain at the slightest stimulus, which ordinarily would be ignored. The brain relates to the gut its own emotional interpretation of the world. Similar events in the gut reinforce that emotional interpretation. Where the two meet there is pain. The messages sent back to the brain give rise to conscious 'gut feelings'. So, IBS is effectively gut feeling gone mad.

CHRONIC FATIGUE SYNDROME

CFS (aka post-viral fatigue) rarely occurs without some of the symptoms of the other conditions we have looked at, such as muscle pain and bowel disturbance. I have learned through experience and research that CFS is just another manifestation of the same thing, so all of the above applies. It is clear to me that fatigue, lethargy and lassitude are simply another way the brain has of protecting itself from danger. It is an emergency defence used to opt out of engaging in things that it perceives to be potentially dangerous or harmful.

Fatigue and pain often go hand in hand as protective mechanisms of alarm and withdrawal. The sufferer adopts fear-avoidance behaviour ('it hurts – that must be bad, so I won't do it' or even 'it will hurt so I won't do it') and they become trapped in the cycle. The wise physician will listen to the story and decide which symptom is most pertinent to treat first, but the basic approach should be the same – find out what the brain has to fear and why, and reverse the strategies it has adopted to protect itself. Then formulate your own bespoke strategy to lead that poor soul out of their suffering.

Before we go further, we need to deal with what I call the 'viral fallacy'. For many years, patients with the symptoms of CFS and fibromyalgia were submitted to a barrage of medical analyses, mainly blood tests. All too often, antibodies to several common viruses were found to be present, most notably Epstein Barr virus, which causes glandular fever, aka 'the kissing disease' (because it was common in teenagers at university), but also shingles (reactivated chickenpox, herpes zoster) and the other herpes strains (cold sores and genital herpes). These viruses were often blamed for the chronic symptoms that recurred. But if you cast your mind back to what I explained about the psycho-neuroendocrine-immunology (PNI) system, you can see why this is misguided. These viruses exist in most of us naturally and sit dormant in the nervous system, waiting for an opportunity to pounce when the host's immune system is depleted or distracted by another infection. Herpes sits in the sensory nerves themselves, where it is prevented from propagating and getting established as an infection by our very efficient immune system until such time as our immune system is suppressed for some reason. In the case of herpes zoster, this will take the form of a shingles outbreak. In most people, it will usually be because of the stress/cortisol effect, in which the circulating cortisol inhibits the immune system. Certainly, our immunity has to mount a response once the virus is active, and in the case of an already fatigued and reduced system, this might be the straw that breaks the camel's back, producing long-term symptoms, such as CFS or fibromyalgia. But it is not the virus itself that causes this; it is the depleted state of the PNI system.

Similarly, auto-antibodies (antibodies against the 'self' that can set up friendly fire) will be found in the blood of people who seem to produce a lot of inflammation in their joints and tissues, but they are also present in many of the population who do not have symptoms.

In the case of students (drinking too much, late nights and working to deadlines) and yuppies (stressful jobs and high-performing, competitive lives), it is hardly surprising that they are susceptible to outbreaks of viruses like glandular fever, herpes and shingles. And, sadly, in an increasingly pressured world, we are seeing younger and younger people falling victim to these conditions. Patients frequently adopt the false premise that they are being attacked by some nasty bug. But the bottom line is, it was the state the patient had got into, caused by all the stressors we have discussed *before* the virus reactivated, that is relevant, not the virus itself.

MIGRAINE

Migraine, a condition that co-exists in up to 50 per cent of fibromyalgia patients, has a similar origin to these other chronic conditions. It starts as increased sensitivity in the primitive brain stem, due to continued fear responses, and spreads as a wave of excitation across the higher cortical centres. As it passes over the key regions of the brain, it produces all sorts of associated visual and auditory symptoms (e.g. scintillations, blind spots and ringing in the ears), as well as nausea and vomiting. For most, the pain is so incapacitating that they shut down and take to their beds. The anxiety that is induced, particularly over the sinister nature of the symptoms and the lack of apparent cure, fuels the vicious cycle.

Once one understands this phenomenon, then the classic distribution of a migraine is predictable. All the parts of the brain involved have a sensory function. Migraine is mediated through the trigeminal nerve, an important cranial nerve that supplies sensation to the face and head. Along with our eyes and ears, it gathers sensory information from our environment around the evolutionarily most important part of the body, the head (after all, it houses the brain). When under attack, the head, neck and face were the most important structures for detecting, sighting and escaping predators. The nerves from them are all hyper-sensitised by the brain, and the state of physiological arousal that is established in 'migraineurs' is constantly raised.

Interestingly, the trigeminal nerve has a very long nucleus, which extends down into the neck section of the spinal cord. From the muscles and joints of the top of the neck, it receives sensory information about where we are in space, and forms an important part of our body-positioning system. This is why atypical migraine can often manifest as pain in the neck rather than in the head and why the visual and auditory symptoms do not occur. Some of my patients ask me why, if migraine is stress-related, they so often get it at the weekend. Migraine experts will tell you that migraine doesn't like change. So, if you are stressed, stay stressed, and if you are not, don't get stressed. This makes sense, because if you are in a constant state of vigilance it is changes in the environment that represent danger. We learn this through our orienting reflex, a clever process by which the brain notices what is different about our world. To an already vigilant and primed migraineur, change is bad.

Another curious fact is that many migraineurs get the symptoms in childhood but it manifests as abdominal migraine (recurrent tummy ache). For some unexplained reason, it converts to headache in their early teens. This is speculation on my part, but I suspect it is because our teens represent the time when we leave the safety of our parents' home and become less vigilant regarding our nurturing and more focused on our new-found need to protect ourselves. Our heads became more important than our stomachs.

GETTING TO THE ROOT OF THE CAUSE

What all these conditions have in common is a state of *physiological hypervigilance*, caused by long-term evolutionary exposure to a multitude of biological, sociological and psychological stressors, to which we have had to adapt and respond. Therefore, to address these conditions, we need to tackle the root causes of our own hypervigilance, as well as our perception of them. Some of the causes we can resolve immediately, as they exist within our current life and lifestyle, for example:

- Lack of education about the problem
- Poor therapeutic relationship with medical team
- Opiate overuse
- Overweight
- Dietary no-nos (e.g. stimulants and sugar)
- Low Vitamin D and B12 levels
- Lack of exercise (the right kind)
- Bad design of working environment
- Poor flexibility and balance

- Inflammation
- Relationship issues (friends, partners and marriage)
- Isolation, loneliness
- Poor job/bad boss
- Repetitive habitual behaviour, both physical and psychological
- Poor sleep patterns (e.g. apnoea)
- Overuse of social media

Some contributing factors are more subtle and potentially more difficult to broach, as they relate to issues from the past, for example early life and upbringing. However, they must still be examined:

- Loss of a parent
- Alcoholism or substance abuse in a parent
- Living with or caring for a sick family member
- Parental catastrophising over health issues
- Single or absent parents
- Emotional detachment from parents
- Narcissistic/manipulative parent
- Rigid religious or cultural upbringing
- High-performing upbringing
- Helicopter parenting
- Early separation a from parent
- Unreconciled adoption
- Post-traumatic stress disorder (can be of subtle origin)

Many of these issues will be beyond the scope of practitioners other than psychiatrists or psychologists. But I've found that helping a patient to recognise the relevance of them and the influence they have on causing and maintaining the problem is a good start. I'm fortunate enough to have good colleagues within the psychological specialties to whom I can refer patients.

Lastly, we have to mention sleep. Fibromyalgia, IBS and migraine sufferers frequently report poor sleep. I have taken it upon myself to read at least five of the best books on sleep for you and have listed them at the back of this book. The only things that none of them seem to go into much depth on as a source of sleep disturbance are stress and anxiety. While I agree that good sleep hygiene (top tips in Chapter 9 later) is vital, because when it is poor it can cause all sorts of problems, I feel it is of little use unless you get to the bottom of what ails the patient in the first place.

Remember: no one has a single answer for all pains, and each person's pain is unique.

You need to find the right team to formulate the right treatment programme for *you*.

The problem for patients is that if they are not lucky enough to find that team, they can end up in what Dr Heidi Prather, head of rehabilitation at Washington University School of Medicine, calls the 'specialty fish pond'. Patients are swimming in a pond of pain and get fished out by one specialty at a time. Each one realises that they can't help so the patient is thrown back, only to be fished out by another specialist, and so on and so on.

In an ideal world, any good pain programme must include a team that can provide physical therapy based on early direct manual techniques to relieve pain as well as gradual physical strengthening to achieve proper body biomechanics and cardiovascular training. Group therapy sessions are also helpful, for help with stress management, sleep hygiene, breathing training and biofeedback. Sometimes cognitive behavioural therapy can help as well.

In the case of fibromyalgia, the right type of exercise, properly graded and paced, is crucial, backed up by good manual therapy. Hydrotherapy in warm water has been proven to be helpful, as has a mixture of aerobic exercise and resistance work. T'ai chi and qi gong are also beneficial and I have many of my patients doing it. Good education releases the fear of pain and allows patients to forge through it. Understand yourself, know yourself and your condition, and move... a lot.

One of the most comprehensive and successful programmes I have observed is at the Cleveland Clinic in the US. Edward Covington, the programme director, said in an online interview: 'The most powerful psychotherapy that the patients receive is in the gym. It is there that they learn to recapture the power of their own bodies, recreate the endurance they lost, and learn to see themselves not as helpless and powerless to deal with their situations but as having the ability to cope physically.' [74]

As far as possible, on Covington's programme, all patients are weaned off their medication. 'The patient comes in cognitively soggy and leaves much clearer,' as one of the team, Judith Sheman, says. 'There are a lot of Kleenex around as patients are made to talk about family dynamics, their fear and miseducation about their pain, as well as their elation over not being told once more, "We can't help you".'

The clinic believes it is essential to help the patient find a new identity beyond that of 'sufferer'.

Sadly, as far as I know, there is nowhere in the UK with

a unit that utilises this approach on such a comprehensive level. And yet we estimate that 43 per cent of the population have a pain problem.

HYPERMOBILITY – A ROOT CAUSE?

In several of the case histories in this book, I have mentioned hypermobility, a condition that is not usually an illness in itself but often causes persistent pain and overlaps with fibromyalgia, CFS and IBS.

More research is necessary to obtain better data, but it seems that about one third of fibromyalgia patients will also be hypermobile. Similarly, a subset of hypermobile patients will develop fibromyalgia, particularly children. It is not always easy to discern which symptoms are from the fibromyalgia and which from the hypermobility, but I will try and give you some pointers

Hypermobility is a spectrum disorder, which means you can range from being mildly double-jointed to resembling Elastigirl or Stretch Armstrong (that shows my age). At the extreme end of the spectrum are two main conditions, Ehlers-Danlos syndrome (EDS) and Marfan syndrome. Like me, you can have Marfanoid traits without having the 'full-monty' condition. Unfortunately, EDS comes with some other nasty problems, which most hypermobile people will never have to worry about.

If you suspect hypermobility is at the root of your pain issues, then I would recommend you visit hypermobility. org. It is the website of one of the world's leading experts on the subject, Professor Rodney Grahame, at University

College London Hospital.

If I had my way, all children would be routinely checked for hypermobility, to provide parents with the right advice and information to help prevent pain in the future. The clinical checks are quick and easy to do and are painless and non-invasive. Even if children are diagnosed, it does not mean they are disabled or unable to lead a full and active life.

Hypermobile joints just have an unusually large range of movement in them. Sometimes, patients describe themselves as very 'bendy', 'loose' or 'double-jointed'. They also notice that they have unusually stretchy skin, as well as stretch marks. Hypermobility is an inherited condition, due to the absence of a gene that produces particular types of collagen in the soft tissues. Collagen is found almost everywhere, especially in the skin, ligaments, muscles, tendons, heart, blood vessels and eyes. Collagen is basically a supportive protein and stiffening agent that helps to hold all our musculoskeletal system together. As they don't have much of it, hypermobile people have to activate their muscles to work harder to help fight against the burden of gravity while also carrying out the usual movements of daily life.

Hypermobility is also commonly associated with lower resting tone in the muscles, and people with it notice they cannot get the same tone and definition in their muscles that other people have, often despite regular exercise. As in fibromyalgia, hypermobile patients tend to produce trigger points in their muscles, which is another reason why the two conditions can overlap or be confused. These trigger points can develop early in life and pre-sensitise them to pain.

The combination of low muscle tone and looser ligaments means that at rest the joints and limbs are poorly supported. This makes you feel stiff because your muscles have to work harder to support the joints. This in turn causes the joints to settle and the joint capsules (the membranes around the joints) to stretch, which ultimately produces pain. As a result, hypermobile children get uncomfortable sitting or standing still for too long and have to shift position. They fidget constantly and jiggle their legs and feet, which adults can find irritating. As I tell patients, they have to move to think. I am a big fan of asking schools to allow hypermobile students to sit at the back and get up and walk around when appropriate, making it clear, of course, that it is not a punishment. In an ideal world, I would give them all standing desks, as children sit too long anyway. There is great evidence that children learn better and are more creative when they can move.

Hypermobile adults also need to get up and move around more often. They are more prone to repetitive-strain-type injuries, and so need to take regular rests from certain tasks.

They also have a tendency to be clumsy; this is not the same as being dyspraxic, which involves poor hand–eye coordination. They are very often flat-footed or get lazy muscles in their feet due to the wrong footwear, particularly shoes that have too much cushioning and not enough support in the uppers. A lace-up is better and should be flexible. They love swimming as it is gravity-free, and the increased extension they have in their knees and shoulders gives them a better stroke. They are also naturally drawn to dancing and gymnastics as they are naturally flexible, and these are the types of exercise that give them the strength and tone they need. So if your child is hypermobile, encourage physical activity early, particularly climbing, balancing and crawling, even if they don't think they are good at it. Martial arts are great, too.

Hypermobile people often complain of pins and needles, numbness and tingling in their limbs. This is because they are more prone to nerves being compressed within the soft tissues under their body weight. Also, there is a significant amount of ligament along nerves, which supports them and protects them from being overstretched. If the ligaments lack collagen, as is the case in hypermobility, they, and the nerves they support, can be stretched more easily.

Low tone in the blood vessels (due to lack of collagen) means that hypermobile people tend to have low blood pressure. Generally, this is a good thing. However, sometimes it makes the vessels respond more slowly to changes in pressure (for example when going from sitting to standing), and people may take longer to adapt to it. This can make them feel faint or dizzy. Occasionally, it is accompanied by harmless palpitations. Hypermobile people are more prone to IBS-type symptoms because the bowel has poor motility and can get inflamed. Girls in particular can get a nervy bladder syndrome, making them feel they need to go more often or more urgently. I am afraid natural childbirth can also permanently stretch the pelvic floor to the extent that even exercises won't help.

Many of my hypermobile patients report that they often feel light-headed in the heat. This is because in hot weather the body tries to cool itself by opening up the blood vessels in the periphery (arms, legs and skin). However, this tends to reduce their blood pressure, which is already quite low, producing a spaced-out feeling. It is harmless but disconcerting.

Weirdly, hypermobile people are more likely to be resistant to the effects of local anaesthetics, such as the ones used in dentistry. They also tend to be vitamin D-deficient and bruise more easily.

What does all this mean? They hurt!

Many people between the ages of 20 and 40 ask me: 'Why have I got all my symptoms *now*?' My answer is that, unfortunately, hypermobility hates inactivity. It hates sitting and it hates habit. When we are fit and well-toned and strong in our teens and early 20s, we do a lot more exercise and are generally more active. Work, on the other hand, tends to involve long hours of sitting and doing the same actions – usually typing on a computer. We just move much less. As a result, our muscles weaken and we slump onto our ligaments, which in the case of hypermobility are weak anyway. The result: sensitisation and pain.

In general terms, the best hypermobility patients are the young, fit, exercising, lean and well-motivated who present with postural problems, muscle strains, tension headaches and occasionally shoulder and knee dislocations. The most difficult to treat are middle-aged, unfit, overweight and deconditioned. But, equally, they are the ones I love to see in clinic because we can mobilise so many different strategies to help them, and when they turn the corner it is very gratifying for all concerned.

As with the other conditions we have looked at in this chapter, explanation and education are paramount to relieve the inevitable anxiety over the distressing symptoms of hypermobility. Many of my hypermobile patients have been relieved and grateful just to have their symptoms linked, diagnosed and explained, so that they can stop being a sufferer and learn to thrive. It immediately empowers them to take the steps to get well and reduce their pain.

The right kind of graded and mixed exercise treats almost all the symptoms, including the cardiovascular ones. Most of my patients start with stretches to specific shortened muscles. These are isometric, postural and balance-based exercises to stabilise their joints in three planes of movement, which are kept simple but should be done daily. The pacing and loading of the exercises is core to their prescription. This is backed up by t'ai chi or qi gong and specific Feldenkrais moves; I rarely advise yoga as people tend to overstretch and we are trying to make them stronger and more stable, not more flexible. After that, they advance quite quickly to more strenuous stuff, with resistance work forming the majority of the programme. As David Butler and Lorimer Moseley, pioneers of pain education, say in *Explain Pain*: 'If you have issues in the tissues, motion is lotion.' [75]

I factor in a series of self-treatment strategies, such as breathing training, body brushing and trigger point release with my Bakpro tools, to relieve inflammation and the contributing peripheral 'feeders' to the pain that lie in the tissues (this calms nociception and changes the type of over-sensitive receptors to less twitchy ones).[76] I am not averse to the use of medication in bad cases, to obtain a window of pain reduction so that patients can get going, but the aim is that they will be completely medication-free by the end of the treatment.

Releasing trigger points – the tender points in muscles that are characteristic of painful musculoskeletal syndromes – with breathing retraining is key. Correct breathing helps to reduce the fear response of the pain and regulate the sensitivity of the points. I also advise my patients to keep well hydrated, eat regularly and not miss breakfast.

Perhaps most importantly, I hold their hands in the early stages but then, once they are ready and can self-manage, I positively reinforce that, in the nicest possible way, I never want to see them darken my door again.

They do occasionally return, because either they have got slack and let things slip, or had a mini-crisis and need to touch base. We reset them and release them once more. As I always tell them, if they need to keep seeing me, I'm not getting them better!

CASE HISTORY: NATHALIE

A talented and articulate woman in her 40s, Nathalie is in great demand on televised discussions and as an expert commentator. Her husband is a wealthy businessman and they have three lovely children, the first conceived by IVF. So far, so blessed. But when Nathalie came to see me, she was at the end of her tether. A fibromyalgia sufferer since her 20s, she had suffered wearying pain for two decades which had now led to grave problems in her marriage. The episodes of migraine that had her bed-ridden once a month wreaked havoc with her schedule, and there were mumblings at work.

Her husband travels constantly, pursuing business projects, and the strain of managing her own work portfolio and the demands of her children, while keeping up a constant battle against the pain, had led Nathalie to take a leave of absence from all employment for six months. She told me in tears that she was fairly sure her husband was seeing other women, who could provide him with light-hearted companionship. She felt anger and guilt over it because, although he was being unfaithful, she somehow understood, as her libido had gone through the floor and they almost never made love. Facing the loss of her marriage and her job, Nathalie was understandably distraught. During our first meeting, she sighed 15 times and held her breath repeatedly.

From shaking her hand on arrival and watching her standing posture, and then noticing her constantly fidget in her seat, with a leg crossed around and inside the other, I realised she was very hypermobile. Although she looked a normal size on television, which famously adds pounds, she was actually painfully thin and poorly muscled from following a wheat-, dairy- and sugar-free diet, which she believed would help control her symptoms. She also tried to avoid red meat, and the protein content in her diet was low.

I listened to her story. Nathalie's father walked out on the family when she was three years old. This memory exacerbated her fears that her own husband would now do likewise: after all, isn't that what men do? She had always sought the affirmation of her father because he was clever and successful. As a child, she had thrown herself into her schoolwork and dance classes and for a time considered professional ballet training. I pricked my ears up at this. Women with hypermobility often excel at ballet. Eventually, though, she had decided on academia because she kept pulling muscles. She remains very active, having swapped ballet for daily yoga and swimming. More clues.

I asked if her mother had ever mentioned whether she crawled as a baby. 'Ha,' she responded. '"Clever Nathalie always does things first" is our family motto.' It was as much family legend that she had walked at 10 months without bothering to crawl as that she was the first in the family to go to university, where she gained a first – obviously!

Nathalie was intrigued when I mentioned hypermobility. It was as if a light switched on when I explained and linked all her symptoms. She resisted, at first, when I told her to give up yoga and swimming and replace them with a specifically targeted, graded regime of weight-training and t'ai chi. I also suggested she reduce her stress response by learning to breathe from her diaphragm and use my tools to release her trigger points and take control of them. I told her she should eat a balanced diet and factor in more protein, otherwise the training would only make her sore, not stronger, and observe a new sleep pattern. Finally, I advised her to work with a good therapist on understanding the impact her father's abandonment of her and the family was still having on her, and possibly why she had serially bad relationships with men.

Always the diligent student, Nathalie threw herself into the new regime, occasionally overdoing it and with the odd wobble in her belief that she could get better but, as a team, we were always there to help her regroup and forge on. By the time her six-month leave of absence from work came to an end, the pain was largely under control. She understood where it was coming from and how to control it if it niggled at her. She was feeling more relaxed and positive than she had for years. The headaches had gone. At our last session, she gave me some surprising news. Still not sure about whether her husband was having affairs, she had, in any case, decided to file for divorce. Her fear of loss of companionship and support no longer outweighed her humiliation at having been cheated. 'What was I thinking? He never supported me anyway.'

CHAPTER 8

THE BREATH OF LIFE

'We are what we repeatedly do.'
– Aristotle

Now, I want to dedicate some space to talking about a process that goes on every second of your existence and to which you probably give no thought at all: breathing. Unless, that is, you have been doing yoga, Pilates or mindfulness, in which case you will have already been introduced to the most fundamental way I know of assessing and improving your health as well as optimising your performance. For the past 25 years it has been at the core of every assessment I have done with patients at my clinic.

Every one of my patients has it drummed into them. I tell them that if they don't do their breathing exercises, there's no point in coming back. That gets their attention! So, if you leave this book with nothing else, just do the exercises I give you in this chapter.

Even if you are pretty sure you've got a handle on breathing – perhaps you have been taught to control yours as a singer or athlete – you will benefit from what I am about to tell you. Elton John, whom I have seen as a patient, calls me 'the man who taught me how to breathe'. Mind you, a famous opera singer who once consulted me about his neck pain was not so convinced at first. When I suggested we take a look at his breathing, he exploded in true operatic fashion: 'For God's sake, man, of course I know how to breathe. Do you know what I do for a living?'

I explained that although he had clearly been trained in the technique of using his diaphragm properly while singing, it was obvious he wasn't doing it the rest of the time. Furthermore, his busy and stressful performance schedule was taking its toll. Some time later he phoned to let me know that not only had his neck pain gone, but he had seen a tonal change in his voice, which he had feared he was losing with age.

Make no mistake, practising the exercises I give you at the end of this chapter for only a few weeks will reward you with astonishing results in both the reduction of symptoms and better constitutional health. Checking that you are staying on track takes just a few minutes and can be done anywhere – at your desk, in meetings, even safely while driving. So, no one has the excuse of saying they are too busy.

〇 〇 〇

Apart, possibly, from the beating of our hearts, breathing is the most important function of the body. It is our only source of our most vital element, oxygen, which we harvest from the air we inspire. The mechanism of breathing is driven by the brain and the nervous and musculoskeletal systems, working in harmony with each other. Receptors all over the body pick up and regulate the oxygen levels in our blood and tissues, paying most attention to the two biggest users of it, our brain and muscles, and constantly adjusting our breathing depth and rate (normally 10–14 breaths per minute at rest) to accommodate the myriad changes that occur in our environments – both internal and external – and which require a subtle alteration in the amount of oxygen we need.

Besides oxygen there's another gas that is critical to our well-being: carbon dioxide (CO_2). This is a by-product of the energy-burning processes in our bodies and needs to be expelled, or expired, at a rate that is consistent with maintaining the correct acid (pH) balance in our blood. When we are stressed, the relationship between breathing in oxygen (inspiration) and breathing out CO_2 (expiration) shifts, and that's where a lot of the problems lie. More on those shortly…

The physical mechanics of breathing rely on the synchronised functioning of the diaphragm, the dome-shaped muscle inside our chests. When we breathe in, it contracts, descends and flattens, allowing air to rush into our lungs with minimal effort. Healthy breathing is slow and deep, flowing rhythmically through the nose, belly and chest. This is how we are designed to breathe throughout our lives. When this pattern is lost, which can happen for a variety of reasons, both physical and emotional, things can start to go wrong. Most of the time we are not aware of our breathing and it ebbs and flows guided by our subconscious breathing centres. But, unlike many of our other bodily systems, we can take conscious control of it.

One of the reasons practising conscious breathing and observing its pattern is so important is that by definition we can only breathe in the 'now' and therefore observing and counting exhalations (the relaxatory bit of breathing) puts us in the present. This is the basis of mindfulness. Like a muscle, it can be honed with training, leading to freedom of thought and focus. The new pattern can become a new 'habit'.

As we saw in Chapter 3, although we may no longer have to worry about sabre-toothed tigers, our modern lifestyle keeps us in a constant low-level flight mode, and if we add in higher levels of emotional trauma such as bereavement, relationship problems, a bad boss, or moving house, then we begin to breathe in the way we might have done when we were being chased across the plains by a predator. Back then, of course, we only had to flee from predators sporadically, after which we could rest, recover and lick our wounds; these days we are exposed to a more constant level of stress – perceived or actual – without periods of recovery.

The trouble is that the sympathetic part of our autonomic nervous system, which governs our 'fight or flight' response, is more active than the parasympathetic part, which controls our 'rest-and-digest' functions. In an ideal world, it should be the other way around. Yes, we should all be as chilled as the sun-kissed surfer 'living the dream', sitting on a board in the gently undulating waves… except we are not, are we?

Everyday stress pushes us more onto the sympathetic side of the see-saw and among other things we begin to breathe in a fight/flight manner – rapidly and shallowly and often holding our breath. This results in an imbalance between the exchange of oxygen and CO^2 across our lungs; we actually 'puff off' too much CO^2, which increases the alkaline in our blood pH levels. (You know the scenes in TV dramas when they give the patient a paper bag to breathe into? This is to recapture the CO^2.) This imbalance between the gases is effectively an alarm state for the brain, known as neuronal hyperexcitability, which immediately reinforces the stress response and causes us to breathe more erratically. In so doing, our 'thinking brain' (the forebrain) shuts down even more, further disabling us from rationalising the anxiety that caused the problem in the first place.

At a mechanical level, poor breathing means we also waste up to 30 per cent more energy a day. This is because instead of using the larger, stronger lower ribs, we begin to recruit and elevate the smaller upper ribs, which goes against gravity and is hard work. In normal breathing, the upper ribs should only be recruited when extra levels of ventilation are necessary, such as during exertion, intense exercise or asthma attacks.

This poor pattern of breathing also leads to significant changes in the posture of the head and neck, as well as increased 'sway' in the low back – the pelvis tilts and the back is overextended, resulting in a misalignment of the entire body. This can induce chest pain, dizziness and pins and needles, and cause you to grind and clench your teeth. Once it becomes a habit, it exacerbates anxiety and affects sleep quality.

The aches and pains arise because certain muscles are made to do increased work for which they were not designed. At least 30 per cent of any neck problem is breathing-related. Over time, muscles develop the painful trigger points we've talked about in earlier chapters. Furthermore, the muscles are forced to store lactic acid (a by-product of the extra muscle metabolism), as it is not excreted through the moisture in our breath during exhalation in the normal way.

Think about when you've been in a stressful environment, and had to participate in a high-pressure meeting or make a presentation. How often have you noticed that you seem to lose your normal degree of articulacy when speaking? That is because as you become anxious about performing, you take faster, more shallow breaths, the cognitive (thinking) forebrain switches off, and your ability to express yourself fluently goes as your more primitive hindbrain kicks in. This is the area related to running away and self-preservation, not talking and debating. Try doing ten long, slow breaths before a difficult meeting; it makes an enormous difference.

Breathing affects everything. Many of my patients who do the breathing training, initially for back or neck pain, for example, can't believe it when I say that it will also help their irritable bowel or constipation symptoms. They just cannot see how they could be linked. As an exercise to convince them, I place a stethoscope over their tummy where the large intestine runs and ask them to tell me what they can hear. The answer is almost always: nothing! What they should hear is the intermittent squelching and squirting noises of peristalsis, the muscular wall of the bowel contracting to propel the digested food along it. I then ask them to carry out ten of the training breaths: long, slow and deep. Usually, within five, the relaxing effect of it stimulates the vagus nerve to activate the digestive processes of the bowel, mainly in the form of better blood supply, enzyme secretion and increased peristalsis. It is also fair to say that some of the noise is the diaphragm descending into the abdominal cavity on the in-breath and pumping the stomach to assist with the mechanical breakdown of the food contents. Even this is advantageous. At their next appointment, if patients have been diligently practising, they almost all report an improvement in their digestive symptoms, including gastric reflux.

There's one more crucial reason for breathing correctly, one you may not have considered: breathing is the only physiological process that gives us access to a psychological state... Or, to put it more simply, breathing is the only bodily process that gives us access to our mental state, and we don't need any expensive equipment to monitor it!

Here's what that means to us in everyday life. When, as humans, we become stressed, we unconsciously activate a series of mental and emotional responses designed to help us decide how to respond to that stress. Long before we consciously realise we are stressed, a whole suite of physiological changes have prepared us for action.

This science forms the basis of the lie detector, or polygraph, test. The operator knows that no matter how hard the subject tries to suppress their natural responses to the stress of telling a lie, the machine finds them out. This is because our 'conscious' brain cannot suppress the physiological responses that our 'unconscious' brain activates. Evolution dictated that any threatening information or circumstances would ready us for action whether we wanted it to or not.

An elegant study carried out in 2009 showed that students wired up to polygraph-style apparatus while using social media on their phones recorded concerning results.[77] All those tested showed significant increases in respiration rate, heart rate and perspiration. A remarkable 83 per cent reported hand and neck pain during texting and held their breath while messaging – although they were unaware that they did so.

I have carried out similar testing myself on a cohort of financial traders at a leading hedge fund, based on a protocol I use every day with my clinical patients. Generally, when traders see volatility in a market, they become stressed – sometimes positively (excitement) and sometimes negatively, if the position they hold is going to be badly affected. Interestingly, however, caught up in the moment, they don't consciously know they are becoming stressed. The downside of stress on traders is that they become risk-averse and do not want to get into a trading position. It can also mean they make bad decisions as a result, because when a person becomes stressed, they shut down their forebrain (the thinking and decision-making parts of the brain), and that's quite scary.

In my study, we attached a breathing monitor to the traders' belts, one that would pick up not only when they began to breathe erratically but also when they either hyperventilated or held their breath – sometimes they did this for up to 30 seconds at a time. Believe it or not, this is common even in people who work in much less intense environments.

Hyperventilation, or hyperventilation syndrome, is the breathing pattern disorder that is responsible for the vast majority of symptoms I see in my patients – symptoms that had doctors in several specialties scratching their heads. It was first identified as a condition in traumatised soldiers as early as 1871 by a military surgeon called Dr Jacob Mendes Da Costa.[78] But it was not until 1937 that William Kerr and his colleagues recognised the relationship between a wide variety of symptoms and 'overbreathing', as they called it.[79] Their research was filed away under psychiatric disorders, because no structural or organic cause was ever found for it.

We now know why that was, thanks to an enlightened 1970s scientist called LC Lum, who conducted various studies on hyperventilation and anxiety and found that, despite its very real impact on the health of sufferers and their capacity to function, hyperventilation syndrome is not a disease… it is a habit.[80] And the habit develops from an initial response to a stressful event, or series of events, initiating a vicious cycle of symptoms that become self-perpetuating and manifest in a number of different ways.

If the hyperventilation goes on for longer than three months, it becomes chronic and the patients will start to show symptoms in all parts of the body, including:

- Frequent sighing and yawning
- Disturbed sleep
- Erratic heartbeat
- Feeling anxious and uptight
- Pins and needles
- Upset gut/nausea
- Clammy hands
- Chest pains
- Shattered confidence

- Fatigue
- Achy muscles and joints
- Dizzy spells or feeling spaced out/foggy-brained
- Irritability or hypervigilance
- Feeling of 'air hunger'
- Breathing discomfort

Any of those sound familiar? Lum went on to say that, as numerous symptoms emerged, the patient's self-confidence began to wane and secondary problems started to develop. Patients would develop a fear of flying or a fear of underground trains, for example, believing that was what was making them feel sick. Sometimes these fears escalated into full-blown phobias. Their anxiety stimulated the stress hormones, causing them to hyperventilate even more.

It truly is a vicious cycle that leads to investigations by specialists – cardiologists, gastroenterologists, neurologists, psychiatrists, respiratory physicians – who, despite carrying out numerous tests, will find nothing abnormal, thus delaying diagnosis for months, sometimes years.

When I worked in primary care, these were the patients who had what we called 'Thick File Syndrome'– they had undergone multiple tests but nothing had ever been found. Ultimately, I realised that the existence of such a file was the clue to the cause.

In some cases, there doesn't even need to be a particularly stressful event to trigger hyperventilation syndrome. Once poor breathing habits have been established and the body has been puffing off carbon dioxide for long enough, it adapts to being depleted and the various receptors change their sensitivity, allowing this to become the new normal.

This removes some of the leeway the body normally has to adapt to further changes, so something as simple as a yawn or a sigh can induce symptoms.[81]

Thus we can see that breathing is intricately related to and tied in with every other system in our body and people who have a breathing disorder as their primary problem will go on to produce a cascade of related symptoms and issues. Equally, people with physical problems will 'express' that dysfunction in their breathing.

When we hyperventilate and the CO_2 levels drop in our blood, an alarm state develops in our brain. This is known as neuronal hyperexcitability and refers to a process by which the nerve cells in the brain become overactive and excitable such that their activity is elevated and the neurones discharge more often and more randomly. There is also an irritational effect induced on them by local circulating inflammatory cells and chemicals (our old friends the cytokines; see pages 91 and 94) often produced by long-term cortisol production. As a result the nerves which communicate the pain we experience also become more sensitive and we perceive this as an elevation in our pain level or intensity. Performing regular breathing exercises returns the CO_2 levels to normal, reversing this effect. It not only reduces the psychological anxiety around the pain but also the pain itself. It calms the 'fearful system' and breaks the cycle.

HOW CAN YOU TELL IF YOU ARE HYPERVENTILATING?

The characteristic signs are sighing, yawning and catching

or holding your breath. Constant tension in the neck and trapezius muscles as well as clenching your teeth at night are also indications. If you snore or have sleep apnoea or breathe through your mouth most of the time, then by definition you are breathing badly. You will probably notice that you have a dry mouth in the morning. It is very important to at least inhale through your nose, if not exhale through it too. Why?

It is because the nose was cleverly designed by nature to be a certain diameter, which helps slow the process of breathing down and increase the amount of time the air has in the lungs to transfer vital gases in and out – gases that include nitrous oxide which helps to lower blood pressure and open blood vessels in the brain.

The nose is also full of enzymes which kill bacteria and viruses. And breathing through your nose passes the air over the adenoids which sit above the back of the throat and which contain immune cells capable of fighting invading infection; while fine hairs in the nostrils catch larger air-borne particles and filter them out.

There is also a network of fine capillary blood vessels in the nostrils, and a large surface area of moist membranes to warm and wet the air as it passes into our airway. If the air is not warm and moist, the deeper airway becomes dry, and reacts by producing mucus to prevent further drying and cracking. It also stimulates mast cells, which are inflammatory and allergenic in their function, to inhabit the area. Many people who have been diagnosed with chronic sinusitis simply have a breathing pattern disorder.

○ ○ ○

So, to summarise the benefits of good breathing:

• It releases muscular tension throughout your body.

• It provides access to and control of your responses to stressful situations.

• It enables you to think optimally when under pressure or in stressful environments.

• It enables you to defuse the fear and protection messages your unconscious mind sends you.

• It improves postural stability: creating a mobile, supportive spine that leads to correct posture, improved balance, fluid movement and agility.

• It improves the health of the nervous system. The brain and nervous system are extremely sensitive to changes in the oxygen and CO_2 balance. The nervous system also houses the spinal column, the circulation to which is pumped by breathing movements.

• It removes waste products: 70 per cent of the body's waste products are eliminated in the breath through exhalation.

• It boosts the lymphatic pump: essential for maintaining the health of the immune system.

• It promotes the 'relaxation response': the conscious use of breathing to induce relaxation and to dispel feelings of anxiety and panic.

• It regulates CO_2 levels (just as important as oxygen levels), and the autonomic nervous system.

• It regulates the body's acid–alkaline (pH) balance,

essential for the optimal functioning of your organs.

SIMPLE STEPS TO BETTER BREATHING

It costs nothing to try proper breathing, so give it a go – it might just change your life. There are various techniques out there, but I have found this to be the most effective, and it's dead easy to remember.

Start with a little test to see whether you are breathing the right way around. You need to check that you do not have an 'inverted breathing pattern', using your neck, pectoral and upper rib muscles to breathe instead of your diaphragm, as described earlier when we talked about hyperventilation.

1. Shut your mouth and give a big sniff.

2. Check what your tummy does. If it is rapidly drawn in towards your spine, then you are breathing the wrong way around. If instead it bellows out and your chest remains motionless, then you are Buddha himself and have already achieved enlightenment and can toss this book away. Sadly, most people will find that the former is the case. Particularly those of you who feel you should hold your tummy in. Don't! Let it all hang out. Otherwise you create the same effect as wearing an Edwardian corset and will be at risk of fainting with the 'vapours'.

3. Now sit in a chair and let the back support you, or even better, lie down with your knees up and feet on the floor. Relax your shoulders and close your mouth. Place your right

hand on your upper chest and your left hand over your navel. For a few seconds monitor your breathing. You will probably notice that your right hand moves first and most. This is the wrong way around.

4. Take a long slow breath in through your nose, imagining that the air is rushing down and into a big balloon in your tummy. As it does so, inflate your tummy, activating your diaphragm to make a pot belly. Also imagine that your right hand has a paralysing effect on your chest, so that you can't use it. If you are doing this correctly, the only thing moving should be your tummy. It may take a few breaths to get it right but don't get frustrated, keep trying. For some people it is changing the habit of a lifetime.

5. Continue that breath in for a count of five. As you get to the end of the in-breath pause for one second and slowly begin to exhale, but for a count of seven this time. Yes, this is longer than the in-breath.

6. Pause for a second at the bottom of the out-breath and again start to inhale for five and so on.

Within five breaths you should notice you are feeling more relaxed and could quite happily shut your eyes. The out-breath is the most important part and is what most people don't do properly. It also activates the vagus nerve to calm the nervous system and switch on all of our rest-and-digest processes. It will begin to clear your thoughts and discourage the negative thought-chatter that is so pervasive when we are stressed. It also immediately coun-teracts the sympathetic drive, which is causing a constant state of internal tension in the muscles – what I call the 'hum'. As described earlier, this wastes energy and causes you to store in your muscles the lactic acid that you would normally excrete, thereby altering the body's pH balance and oxygen levels.

Repeat this exercise ten times and then return to a normal and natural depth of breathing but continue to make sure it is coming from your tummy and not your chest. If you do more than ten breaths, you may feel a little light-headed. This is normal and will pass; it is just that you are not used to this amount of gas exchange in your lungs. In fact, it shows how you have got used to faulty breathing.

The more you practise, the less this shallow breathing will happen. I ask patients to commit to five sessions of ten breaths per day. As soon as your eyes open, do ten before you get up. Ten in the mid-morning, ten in the afternoon and ten when you get home and a last set lying in bed before sleep. It has a profound effect on sleep, optimising your recovery-type sleep.

If you catch yourself sighing, yawning or holding your breath during the day, do five correction breaths to reset.

To recap: mouth closed, nose only... in for five seconds... out for seven seconds... Repeat ten times. Five sessions a day if possible.

Yes, it really is that simple and, as in the words of the great 1970s Martini advertisement, it can be done any time, any place, anywhere.

If you want to develop your breathing further you can try these subtle variations:

3-4-5 BREATHING

This is very good for people who are prone to anxiety or stress. It is great to do at work if you can find a quiet spot or even at your desk. Breathe in (ideally, with your mouth closed) for three seconds, hold for four seconds and breathe out for five seconds. Simple. Do this for five minutes if you can, or even a few rounds before a stressful meeting, event or presentation.

BOX BREATHING

This is great to do before bed and put you in to recovery sleep. Breathe in for four seconds (again, mouth closed), hold for four seconds, breathe out for four seconds and hold for another four seconds.

ALTERNATE NOSTRIL BREATHING

This is a really good exercise for deep relaxation and to train yourself to breathe through your nose and not your mouth, as well as to clear sinusitis. It is very energising.

It is known as *Nadi shodhan* by the yogis and has been practised for centuries.

Once you are sitting or lying comfortably, place your thumb over your right nostril and block it. Fully exhale through your left nostril. Breathe in through your left nostril for a count of four seconds.

Now block your left nostril and breathe out through the right one for four seconds. Then breathe back in through the right nostril for four seconds. Block the right nostril again and breathe out through the left one. You have completed one cycle. Repeat ten cycles.

Try it; you will not regret it.

CHAPTER 9

TOWARDS A PAIN-FREE FUTURE

'It is not the curse or blessing that works, but the idea.
The imagination produces the effect.'
– Paracelsus

Having come this far on the journey with me, you may
by now used to expecting the unexpected. If so, good!
Because now I want to introduce you to the most exciting new developments in pain relief, which consist
not of clever new drugs, but of fewer drugs, or even none
at all.

I'm going to tell you about the fascinating phenomenon
of the placebo. Medical professionals are generally tentative
about its use, as if it were in some way a tool of the dark
arts. But, for me, it represents a combination of the summation of therapeutic experience and the confirmation of
the existence of nature's medicine chest.

THE PLACEBO EFFECT

A placebo is an inert drug or treatment that is administered to the patient; and the placebo effect is the outcome of that treatment or drug, seen as a change in the condition of the patient's symptoms. The important fact is that the placebo is an unknown entity. It is an effect, not a thing. This very definitely does not mean that you can just take something that tastes or feels nasty, is expensive or difficult to obtain, wrap it up in mystery and call it a cure.

Traditionally, doctors have been forbidden from using the placebo effect to treat their patients, as it contravenes their ethical promise. This is because it was seen in some way to be duping or deceiving the patient. It went against the belief that the patient had the right to be informed fully about the treatment and its possible side effects, and consent to it.

In the case of placebo, you would be forgiven for thinking that side effects were an impossibility, of course, as the drug is inert. However, research has shown that if patients believe they are receiving a drug, then, despite it being a sugar pill, they will present with many of the drug's side effects anyway. Furthermore, they will go through the symptoms of withdrawal when they stop taking it. This confirms that much of the effect is down to the power of belief alone.

The placebo effect has been calculated across many studies to account for anything between 30 per cent and 50 per cent of the response to a range of drugs.[82] One outlier was antidepressants, the placebo for which was 79 per cent effective. That is pretty extraordinary! As a result of this discovery, researchers are having to factor the placebo effect into their studies, to ensure that the drug is more effective than the placebo. Studies have shown that the simple act of taking a drug creates elements of expectation and conditioning, perception, confidence, need and want in the patient. In experiments, some people believed that a more expensive 'painkiller' was more effective than a cheaper one, despite both being no more than sugar pills. Others reported that a more expensive sports drink relieved their fatigue more effectively than another.

I have found in my own patients that more expensive, branded drugs are perceived to be more effective than cheaper generic ones, even though they contain exactly the same active ingredients and formula. Drug companies will never admit it publicly, but this is why they colour-code tablets according to what they contain. They knowingly use the placebo effect to enhance the effect of the drug. Have you ever noticed that painkillers are usually white, anti-inflammatories yellow, pink or red, and antibiotics multicoloured capsules? Research has shown that the colour of the pill enhanced outcome when it contained only sugar.[83] So, if you are running a commercial enterprise, why wouldn't you capitalise on the advantage? The language and the visuals on the box are all designed to create maximum effect.

Conditioning, as well as belief, is involved in this response. An experiment carried out in 2009 showed that a sweet tablet given to lower the immune systems of mice was just as effective when they removed the active ingredient and left only the sweetener.[84] The mice had learned to associate sweetness with a required effect. Another study made a similar finding in humans.[85] The researchers gave medication to individuals with a dust-mite allergy and asked them to take it with a 'special' drink. When they replaced the drug with a placebo, the subjects saw just as good a reduction in their allergic symptoms as when they took the drug. However, they saw no improvement when the placebo was given with water. The 'special drink' had produced a conditioned response. So we can see that the placebo effect is not confined to the realms of pain. The brain is capable of mounting all sorts of internal mechanisms, its own 'medicine chest', when it wants to.

Surprisingly, the effect extends to surgery, too. In 2002, an American team of researchers constructed a study to examine the effectiveness of arthroscopic surgery for painful knee conditions.[86] They wanted to see whether it altered the natural evolution of the condition. Some 180 patients were told that they would either have a regular arthroscopic knee operation, a simple washing-out of the joint with saline, or a sham operation (where no procedure at all was carried out). In order to convince all the patients that they had had surgery, small incisions were made in the skin to mimic those made in a real operation.

All the patients were monitored for two years after the surgery. At one stage, the placebo group was doing better than the other two groups who had undergone the real procedure, and in the end the outcomes for all three groups were about the same. Amazing!

○ ○ ○

Even the nature and structure of the healthcare system

has its effect on the patient's belief system. A study in 2017 showed that a third of Americans and Australians had reported feeling pain often or very often in the past month.[87] This was in startling contrast to China at 19 per cent, South Africa at 11 per cent and just 8.5 per cent in the Czech Republic. The reasons for this are not entirely clear; certainly, the subjects' nervous systems are no different. But the researchers established that it seems to depend on the societal expectations of the national healthcare system concerned. If the system is good and, perhaps more importantly, free, people quickly expect to be pain- and disease-free; after all, it is their 'right' as consumers. Thus, their tolerance for pain or disease is lowered and a feeling of loss for the health they should expect ensues. This manifests as an escalation in their pain. Furthermore, if the health system fails to deliver the expected outcome, this effect is magnified by a sense of loss *and* injustice, resulting in more pain. I suspect this is a key element in the overloading of our NHS service in Britain.

Thanks to the wonders of functional magnetic resonance scanning, we can test the placebo effect by looking at which part of the brain lights up when a drug or placebo has been administered. As I explained in Chapter 2, the two key areas involved are the amygdala, responsible for processing the emotional element of the stimulus, and the hippocampus, which is responsible for memory. We can deduce, therefore, that it is likely that the amygdala is where belief lies and that the hippocampus is responsible for conditioning, as it requires memory to 'remember' the associated response necessary. Another region, the nucleus accumbens, also comes into play. It is associated with pleasure and reward and thought to be the area involved in addiction. It would seem that when this is activated it floods with our old friend dopamine and creates pleasure. A similar effect occurs with a placebo. The pleasure centre lights up with the *expectation* of reward, not just the reward itself.

The piece of research that rocked the placebo boat and indeed, medical research generally, was by Ted Kaptchuk, professor of medicine at Harvard Medical School.[88] He wanted to see if it mattered whether people knew that what they were taking was a placebo. He openly gave placebos to people with irritable bowel syndrome, while reinforcing the point that placebos had been shown to produce self-healing processes. The research team was gobsmacked to find that even when the drug was clearly marked 'placebo' it still had a marked effect on their symptoms. This showed that, despite knowing the drug was inert, the level of expectation and belief were such that it still produced the internal responses they needed.

In my view, this has loosened the ethical confines used to prevent doctors offering an element of placebo within their management of a patient. I, for one, freely admit that I try to maximise the patient experience (I guess we could call this expectation) from the moment they arrive at my clinic door; from the ride in the lift to being greeted at the reception desk. I like to think that at each step of their journey through the building they receive subliminal messages that they are in a place of healing, which will deliver its service in a confident, professional and empathic way, and which will take them and their condition seriously. I try to instil this in everyone who works in the clinic and in my students. If patients arrive in the consulting room with the subconscious mindset of 'I really feel I could get better here', then we have won half the battle. I want the effect of our treatment and advice to ride on the back of any placebo effect we have created before we start. Even the language we use in the clinic has an impact. For example, patients in pain often use words of conditionality and negativity, such as 'would', 'could' or 'if'. If you couch any responses in terms of 'will', 'can' and 'going to', their language changes too, as does their attitude to the potential for recovery. This translates as hope. We try to turn them into *possibilitarians*, on the basis that seeing the possibility of recovery makes the probability of it much more likely.

One frustrating way in which modern medical services further reduce the chances of the combined effect of treatment and placebo is by removing patient choice. In the UK, patients can choose neither their GP nor the consultant they see if they are referred to hospital; they are referred to a team, not an individual. Even in the private sector in the UK, medical insurance companies have begun to set themselves up as the arbiters of whom the patient can see, very often recommending not who is best but who is cheapest. If, as we have already discussed, part of the placebo effect is based on a belief mechanism, then removing patient choice also reduces their belief in the doctor they have been allocated. In an ideal world, people would get to choose who they want to see based on the personal recommendations of friends, family or their GP. Getting a referral by reputation is key to the success of the doctor, too, as it 'preloads' the patient with good expectations and an anticipation of being healed, even before they arrive for their appointment.

Professor Kaptchuk put it well in a TED talk in 2014, explaining that for too long we have ignored placebos as if they were a distraction from pure hard science. Researchers have felt that they are being tasked with finding a precise pharmacological solution to an illness; that science is where the answers lie. Placebos are just fluffy stuff that is hard to quantify and so the 'art of medicine' has been neglected.

But placebo studies take the tools of medicine and change the art of medicine into the science of clinical care. They demonstrate that the human dimension of providing healthcare can alleviate symptoms and change the course of illness even without pharmaceuticals. This does not mean that we want to do away with pharmaceuticals. Placebos cannot shrink tumours, nor can they lower cholesterol, but they can be used effectively to make a good drug or treatment a better one. And there is no better purpose for this than the treatment of pain, in which, as we have seen, emotions, fear, expectation and conditioning play such a crucial role. What we need to envision is a healthcare system that rebalances good medicine with good human care.

OK, I hear you saying, I don't want a cosy chat with a practitioner. I'm in pain and I want strong drugs to stop it. I hear you, and in the short term, of course, we should use drugs, to get patients over the hurdle of acute injury, or post-operative or cancer pain, but they should have little or no place in the treatment of persistent pain. The problem is that all drugs produce side effects and the crisis created by the overprescription of opiates, particularly in the US, has reached catastrophic proportions. It is not as if it is a new phenomenon; opiates in the form of morphine, used to treat the wounded in the American Civil War, left 400,000 soldiers addicted to it. But time has the capacity to fade the memory. Between 1999 and 2017, 200,000 Americans died of opiate overdose. It is believed it will take 60 years for the effects of opiate addiction to wash through society. Tragically, 90 per cent of the addicts walking the streets have no history of drug problems; they are people who had pain and were prescribed these medications. Once they could not get repeat prescriptions from doctors, they had to resort to street dealers to get relief, and the cycle of addiction began. Unfortunately, in people addicted to opioids, the pain itself gets worse rather than better, due to a phenomenon called opioid hyperalgesia. This is when the receptors become more sensitive as the drug wears off and so they need more and more to achieve the same effect. It is similar to the stress-induced hyperalgesia I mentioned in Chapter 3.

There is a closer connection between opioid drugs and the natural placebo effect than you might imagine. Most of the placebos that have an effect on pain do so by stimulating the release of our own internal opiate-based painkillers. Receptors for these chemicals can be found throughout the brain, brain stem and spinal cord, hence their having far-reaching effects, not only centrally in the brain but also on early reception of potentially pain-inducing signals from the body. The effect of placebo on these receptors was initially proven by using an agent (naloxone), which blocked the receptors from the opiates and eradicated the effect of the placebo. These receptors are particularly abundant in the parts of the brain that process emotional feelings. This is why if you ask a badly wounded soldier if he still feels pain after the administration of morphine, he will reply: 'Yes, I still feel pain but I just don't seem to care.'

It is this emotional blockade that is at the heart of the addictiveness of opiate medications. They remove the emotional bridge that links the primitive drives of the brain stem with the higher, more rational and thinking centres of the cortex. Rather than blocking pain itself, the drugs lift the patients out of themselves and away from their interpretation of their pain. In so doing, they remove not only the physical but also the emotional suffering, seeming to dissolve the conflict between the person's desire to live a meaningful life and the reality of their circumstances. Thus they become dissociated from their life, and they withdraw from it. 'No suffering' is effectively the same as pleasure, neurologically speaking.

One can rage at the pharmaceutical companies that developed these drugs and marketed them as safe, but the genie is out of the bottle now. And the net effect of the opiate crisis in the US is that Big Pharma is in no hurry to repeat those mistakes, and the development of more powerful pain-relieving drugs has for the most part been shelved, not least because they don't make them enough money. You may not like the idea that the way to a pain-free future lies largely in your own hands and those of a good practitioner whom you trust, but there is no silver bullet that is going to relieve you of that responsibility any time soon.

This brings us to the importance of trust in the therapeutic experience. In his fascinating book, *The Patient's Brain*, Professor Fabrizio Benedetti addresses this subject, breaking down the experience of seeking therapy into four main steps:[89]

1. Feeling pain: this occurs through sensory information from the body (bottom-up) modulated by how the patient feels about it (top-down).

2. Seeking relief: this is where motivational and reward mechanisms are initiated to seek relief of discomfort. Presentation to the therapist follows.

3. Meeting the therapist/doctor: here the healer must incite trust and hope for there to be a positive response in the patient. This should be met with compassion and empathy by the therapist. Placebo effect begins.

4. Receiving the therapy: the therapeutic act activates expectation and further placebo mechanisms as well as anxiety reduction.

If all these experience mechanisms are positive and they incorporate a bio-psycho-social approach, the therapy/placebo combination is not only maximised but has the power to do great things.

To give just one example of how important the patient–doctor relationship is, we can look at trust as an active ingredient of that relationship. Trust is in fact *the* most important thing for a patient to feel towards a therapist. To be trustworthy, the practitioner must meet five requirements: competence, compassion, confidentiality, reliability and communication. No pressure there then!

The brain is capable of making decisions on trustworthiness very quickly indeed, probably because, for our ancestors, detecting how trustworthy someone was was essential for survival. In fact, just 100 milliseconds (one tenth of a second) of exposure to a face is enough for the brain to decide. That is quicker than the human eye can move around the face to scan it. Who said first impressions don't matter?

Hope is the other key determinant of response to therapy. It has been shown to help patients to tolerate pain for longer and to adjust better to coping with it. Hopelessness has been linked to depression, as it implies a negative expectation of the future. Its partner, helplessness, can be seen as an individual's unrealistically low impression of their own capabilities. The more dangerous version, *learned helplessness*, occurs when attempts at self-help have failed multiple times and the belief that all is lost has set in. With the right approach, both of these states can be prevented or at least improved through the whole therapeutic experience.

So, I hope you can see that understanding the field of placebo is vital to the whole patient experience and that we should not be afraid of using it. Practitioners should be busy factoring it into, rather than out of, their clinical work, while being mindful of its power to confuse and, of course, being honest in their intent.

There is something rather wonderful about Dr Frank Vertosick's statement that 'just as the source of suffering lies in humanity, the cure may be found in our humanity also'.

RAISING RESILIENT CHILDREN

I have already explained why modern life, with its lack of activity and plethora of artificially induced stressors, is leading us towards a more painful future. Along with all the other problems that children will inherit from us, such as global warming, this is their destiny – unless we take positive steps to give them the necessary skills and resilience to minimise its impact. Resilience should not mean, as it has come to in some corporate circles, that you simply reframe stress and bottle it up.

If you have children, or even if you work with children, you will understand the heart-wrenching agony you feel when they are in pain. The desire to take it away from them is all-consuming. Even a simple fall in the playground makes you want to swoop over, sweep them up and reassure them. And this interaction between the carer and the child is vitally important in the development of their pain responses in later years. The mutual transference of the experience of suffering makes up part of what it is to be human.

Imagine that your daughter has just tripped and fallen on the tarmac surface at the swings. For a split second she evaluates what has happened, a rude interruption to her happy play. A brief look of utter shock and surprise. If she can see you, she assesses your response too. Is your face also shocked and horrified? Is it reinforcing her own notion of whether to scream and panic? Or is she greeted by a benevolent grimace and the reassuring low tones of 'oh dear... upsy daisy', as you rush forward to dust her down with a flurry of distractive physicality, designed to desensitise her to the hot burning pain of grazed knees and hands that wants to flood her nervous system, and not give her time to consider and catastrophise?

If you have a deeper interest in this subject, I would highly recommend you read Judy Foreman's excellent book, *A Nation in Pain*.[90] Foreman cites evidence which suggests that children who have been exposed to painful events, but who are treated with a subtle mix of concerned love and a large pinch of reassurance, distraction and physical comfort, such as a hug, manage pain in the future much better. Parents on the other hand who take a 'suck it up' attitude and offer little or no physical solace and those who over-respond and catastrophise over small injuries tend to produce adults with low pain thresholds or dysfunctional responses to their pain or the pain of others.

Obviously, a case can be made for the use of drug-induced pain relief when it is acute and needs relieving. Believe it or not, for many years, quite major surgery was carried out on children without any form of pain relief. Doctors believed that if surgery was necessary to save a child's life, they should carry it out immediately and that the child probably wouldn't remember it anyway. And, since they did not know how to anaesthetise babies, they had to believe they couldn't feel pain. Several paediatric consultant anaesthetists whom I have interviewed have backed up these facts. Babies were routinely given paralysing agents but no pain relievers to block the peripheral pain signals, which meant that, although they could feel pain, they could not move, cry, or in any way indicate that this was so. However, it was evident they were in pain because it was reflected in the monitoring of vital signs, such as blood pressure, pulse rate and oxygen requirements, which would routinely skyrocket due to pain-induced stress hormones being released into the bloodstream.

Shocking though it may seem, until recently there has been little research into how children process pain, and it is still poorly understood. One of the first recognised papers into the undertreatment of pain in children was published in 1975 by PhD student Joann Eland at the University of Iowa.[91] The paper transformed pain intervention for children in her own hospital, but it took years for this to be replicated elsewhere. Survey studies carried out in the 1980s showed that children were not at the time routinely given pain relief during painful procedures, even for full operations and burn debridement, an incredibly painful procedure, in which dead layers of skin are scraped from burns.

It was only when research into the neurobiology of brain development in children proved that babies and children did indeed feel pain that the medical world changed its view and recognised that pain management was paramount.

Pain researcher Maria Fitzgerald published several seminal papers in the UK, which tracked the postnatal growth of pain pathways and the changes that occurred in them under the assault of severe pain.[92] She also importantly showed that local painkillers could reduce the risk of subsequent chronic pain, and that untreated pain in children could have long-term adverse effects.

In 1987, American scientists Anand and Hickey showed unequivocally that human newborns have the anatomical and functional components required for the perception of painful stimuli.[93] Therefore, there was every reason to believe that children could have the same pain experiences as adults, if not as learned and modified.

During the process of birth itself, it is clear that babies are actively trying to manage pain. Even if the birth is relatively easy for the baby (Caesarean or quick vaginal delivery), it pumps into its bloodstream three to five times the level of endorphins (painkilling chemicals) that adults do at rest. Breech or forceps deliveries often produce even higher levels. Nature clearly gave them the means by which to handle this natural process.

It is certainly true that the use of anaesthesia and opiates in children carries greater risk than in adults, but that does not mean that we should not use them. It simply means we have to learn more about them as a specialism and develop better techniques, and also be more discerning about when we perform invasive procedures in the first place. The use of opiate drugs in treating children in pain has now been extensively tested and very little of concern has been found regarding their addictiveness, unlike in adults. Nor is there justified concern about the side effect they have of reducing breathing rate, provided they are handled by specialists.[94] In fact, it has been clear for some time that children who receive good pain relief during surgery do better than those who do not. Yet we still use them far too little. Things are improving, but very slowly. It is only through pressure from the patient body, as well as doctors and nurses, that we can create a movement for change.

Fortunately, there are other non-drug-related approaches that we can use to relieve milder pain in children, such as, curiously, using things that taste sweet.[95] Professor Celeste Johnston of McGill University cites the simple practice of extracting blood with a needle from a newborn's heel to draw blood for testing, as an example. This commonplace procedure, she points out, is 'size-wise, like a knife in the foot of an adult'; i.e. the size of the needle wound relative to the size of the child's foot is equivalent to the extent of the injury to the nervous system. Amazingly, giving them something that tastes sweet when the blood test is performed, in the form of sugar or even artificial sweetener, significantly reduces the length of time that the newborn cries due to the pain of the needle. It is suggested that the sugar works by acting on opioid receptors, and this has been supported by the fact that mothers who are dependent on methadone (the controlled liquid version of heroin) produce children who do not benefit from the sugar response. This is because all the opioid receptors are already full and further relief cannot be stimulated.

Other more innocent approaches, such as dummies and breastfeeding, have been shown to help control minor pain. But interestingly, the best infant pain reliever, which probably comes to parents most naturally, is close, skin-to-skin contact and cuddling. This type of intervention, if we must call it such, which brings together the child and parent or carer or even protector, is born of a natural response to relieve the fear in and danger to the infant that may ensue from a potentially painful stimulus. To me it shows that intrinsic systems exist within our nervous system to link pain to a 'fear and protection' response and that these begin very early in our development.

OVER TO YOU...

We all need to look for ways to help us move out of the pain paradigm. Perhaps more than anything, we need to develop the capacity to deal with our own feelings and desires to protect ourselves from illness and pain. Psychologists call this 'emotional competence'. Certainly, in almost all my persistent-pain patients, this is the element that is most often compromised. We need to foster it in our children as the best preventive medicine. Gabor Maté cites Ross Buck's list of the requirements for emotional competence as follows:

- The capacity to feel our emotions, so that we are aware when we are experiencing stress.

- The ability to express our emotions effectively and thereby to assert our needs and to maintain the integrity of our emotional boundaries.

- The facility to distinguish between psychological reactions that are pertinent to the present situation and those that present residue from the past. What we want and demand from the world needs to conform to our present needs, not to unconscious, unsatisfied needs from childhood. If distinctions between past and present blur, we will perceive loss or threat of loss where none exists.

- The awareness of those genuine needs that do require satisfaction, rather than their repression for the sake of gaining the acceptance or approval of others.

If we accept that many of the issues contributing to pain are rooted deep in the unconscious, from the past as well as the present, then maybe that is where we should go looking and we need to change the way we see our current environment too. After all, we know that a large part of the placebo effect (in pain relief) is mediated through the activation of our own internal opiate and dopamine systems, so we need to find a way of inducing it in ourselves.

Shawn Achor is a psychologist, happiness researcher and author at Harvard. He is the founder of GoodThink,[96] and has made amazing inroads into showing how happiness is achievable and how it can improve our lives immeasurably. He posits that most of us judge ourselves by how the average set of the population behaves and achieves. By definition, the average is only at the 50th percentile of the population. We forget that everyone else within the 'bell curve' above or below that line is still normal, just not average. The lens through which we see the world shapes our reality and the reality in which we live defines us. He asks how you can see the possibility of success or happiness if, in the mindset in which you sit, neither is possible.

We need, therefore, to change our reality. Achor quotes the interesting fact that every second of our lives our brains are confronted with 11 million pieces of information. Yet our brains can only process this information at 40 bits per second. Thus, we have to choose our reality based on the bits that we process. Technically, we can choose to change our reality.

Achor wants us to reverse the way we see the route to success. For most of us, happiness will come with the achievement of success, as in 'when I am more successful, I will be happier'. So, we work harder and harder and then, when we achieve that success, we simply move the goal posts and change what success looks like. Ergo, we are never happy, only exhausted. We need to reverse the formula for success, for it undergirds our parenting and managing styles, and the way that we motivate our behaviour. If we are positive in the present, the brain floods with dopamine, which not only makes us happier but also turns on all our learning centres and changes the way we see the world. In the case of pain, it motivates us to change and allows us to see the possibility of getting better. If we can see happiness as the joy we get from achieving our potential, then we are halfway there. Achor cites five strategies for achieving this mindset:

- Showing gratitude: by writing down three things you are grateful for each day for 21 days.

- Reliving a positive experience: by journalling about something that has made you feel good over the past 24 hours.

- Doing exercise: to teach your brain that your behaviour matters and release opiates and dopamine into it.

- Practising mindfulness: to free your brain from our stressful world.

- Performing random acts of kindness: this can be something as little as opening your inbox and emailing someone in your social network and thanking or praising them for something they have done.

Such mindset changes allow us to give value and meaning to activities and encounters and help us to move forward. We feel more attuned to assuming responsibility and taking on challenges and gaining the self-esteem of achieving them. Even more importantly, as role models to our children we have to send such messages through our behaviour.

This is all about knowing ourselves better, as having such insight facilitates change. Yuval Harari, author of the wonderful book *Sapiens*, recently made this point in an interview.[97] He said that if we are going to use technology and let it into our lives, we have to know ourselves more than ever; for, if we don't, the tech companies will begin to remove our free will by hacking us – something I think a lot of us feel is already happening. They don't have to understand the human brain very well, just build algorithms that know us better than we do. Then they can predict and manipulate our decisions and make choices on our behalf; and that would be very bad for us. We would become reliant on others, feel disenfranchised and powerless, stop taking responsibility and rely on the state to tell us what to do.

As long ago as the 1970s, BF Skinner discovered that media companies used a phenomenon called the Variable Reward Schedule to get us addicted to what we watch.[98] It turned out that it is the *inconsistency* of the reward that sucks us in. If it is predictable we get bored. Therefore, with modern social media we need to check in all the time. James Williams, former Google advertising strategist and now Oxford philosopher, implores us to take back control in our relationship with tech.[99]

As information becomes more plentiful and floods our minds, the resource that is becoming ever more scarce is our attention. He describes what he calls the 'Attention economy', in which media and advertising companies are not on our side and are battling for our attention. As a result, we are so busy with 'stuff' that we stop achieving our own personal goals and never move forward.

The last point I want to make here is regarding our beloved British health system. It is our responsibility to respect and look after it. It is still the finest in the world and driven by amazing people. But we drive it harder and harder with more demands and constant criticism. Personally, I believe that we should not simply pump more and more money into it but take a harsh look at how we as citizens are using it and accept that there are some things we have to fund ourselves, or take steps to treat ourselves, and try to lead a healthier life.

Pain treatment, for one, could move out of hospitals entirely, if we operated a polyclinic-type system in large regional health centres where a multidisciplinary pain team could work in tandem with teams of primary-care professionals. Pain training should be part of all medical degrees; currently, the average time spent on the subject in a doctor's degree is about an hour. Such integrated planning is the future, with communities reconnecting with and looking after each other. It could be an exciting time, too, for architects and planners to fundamentally change the buildings in which we work, once more engaging us with our environment and encouraging collaboration as well as facilitating regular movement.

It is happening, but just takes time.

THE SELF-HELP BIT

This book is not meant to be a detailed step-by-step guide to easing whatever pains you. It could never be that. The reasons why each individual is suffering are too complex for that. Rather, it is designed to set you thinking about what your body is trying to tell you through the hard-to-interpret medium of pain – and how to go about listening. That said, I would be remiss if I didn't mention some of the basic things that I would talk you through if you showed up in my clinic. Your personal lifestyle healthy habits will keep your pain away much better than any trip to a doctor. For many it will be enough.

NB: This advice is for sufferers of persistent pain that has lasted more than three months – people in whom all the tissue damage should have healed but the top-down processes are still in play. It's not for acute pain after injury or trauma.

1. **Accept that the answer rarely lies in a medical prescription, unless there is an established inflammatory process going on.** Your doctor should be the judge of that. The side effects of opiate drugs can end up being worse than the pain itself. Dosage should be strictly monitored. I make an exception here for post-surgery or cancer pains, for which opiates can work very well. Otherwise use over-the-counter pain relief such as ibuprofen or paracetamol, provided you can tolerate them and you follow the instructions.

2. **Don't wait to get help.** No one will give you a medal for waiting until the pain is unbearable. Express it to people

and let them know you are struggling, but with a view to doing something about it rather than complaining and doing nothing.

3. **Be honest with yourself.** This is a hard one. Look deep into yourself and ask whether what you are seeking is what we call in the trade secondary gain from your pain. This is where, whether or not we like to admit it, there is an advantage to having and being incapacitated by pain. For example, do you get looked after more and have to do less? If you live on your own, is it an inadvertent way of getting attention from your family and friends? The answer is to address the cause, not the pain.

4. **Apply the bio-psycho-social test.** Once it is established that your pain is chronic, you need to review the biological, social and psychological elements to understand why your brain is persisting in sending danger messages when the immediate crisis has passed. This is best done with a qualified practitioner whom you trust and who will ask the right questions. Doing it yourself means you will miss key elements; it is difficult to be objective as the patient.

5. **Find a good osteopath or physio.** It is also the case that lack of activity or unbalanced movement caused by a painful episode (such as past trauma) can lead to biomechanical asymmetries and produce trigger points or shut down muscles. This can produce great discomfort but can easily be released or 'woken up' by a good osteopath or physiotherapist, or even home techniques, giving almost instant relief.

6. **Keep moving.** Bed rest is very rarely the answer and the muscle wastage caused by even a couple of weeks of inactivity will compromise your healing and embed the pathways in

your brain that say you are 'broken'. Again, a good osteopath, physio or well-qualified personal trainer can help you
explore safe ways to extend your range of movement in a
paced and graded way.

7. **The best forms of exercise** are walking, running, swimming and cycling (depending on your age and fitness level)
for cardiovascular health; multidirectional or functional
weight training (to improve muscle tone); and t'ai chi for
balance and flexibility – also essential for a healthy old
age. As I have stated, hypermobile patients love yoga and
dance, where they can show off their flexibility, and swimming because it renders them weightless. But these activities won't make you better unless you combine them with
resistance exercise, such as weights. Get a programme built
for you by someone who knows what they are talking about.
Unbalanced training is worse than none at all. Hydrotherapy
is awesome and can be in your local pool, with exercises
from your physio or osteo or some good apps. The warmer
the water the better. Once you have plateaued, move out of
the water to floor exercises and standing balance exercises.

Pilates can be marvellous or terrible, depending on how it
is taught. If it is taught well, it can produce a strong core that
helps every other aspect of your health, but I see so many
people in my clinic who have been taught badly or attend
classes that are too large. They also never migrate from floor
work. Always go to a physio-led class and get a personal or
professional recommendation.

8. **If you work at a desk for much of the day, get a proper
ergonomic assessment of your position.** If possible, install
a standing desk and change your posture frequently – the
best posture is the next posture. If not, get up and walk

around at least once an hour. Do stretches at your desk and engage others to do so. Create your own culture, even if it isn't your company's. If you are on the phone, pace, don't sit. Don't eat lunch at your desk; go out. Beware of what I call the laptop-latte position I see in every coffee shop and communal work space, where the user is curled over a laptop on a low table. You might think you are just checking a few emails but you can easily pass an hour or more in that awkward position. If you use a laptop, put it on a desk and use a laptop stand. Don't cross your legs at your desk or in meetings. And use the stairs… always. Easier is not the path to progress.

9. **Drink water regularly** and put an electrolyte tablet in the bottle every so often to make sure you don't leach out the good chemicals you need.

10. **Be sensible about heavy bags.** I see too many women with their bodies pulled out of natural alignment by a stuffed shoulder bag. The worst of all are the trendy large totes that only work over a shoulder. A properly fitting rucksack and supportive trainers should be your default for commuting.

11. **The shoe conundrum.** The human foot is designed to move and to be in contact with the floor as much as possible, so shoes are effectively sensory deprivation devices for feet. That said, we have adapted somewhat to them and it is too late to change for most, particularly as we get older. If you want the best of both worlds Vibram and Vivobarefoot soles are great and there is a gathering number of styles out there (though they will not be to everyone's taste). Heels if you are used to them, ladies, are not as bad as people think. So wear them, but for short periods, and not at work. During the day an inch is enough. Don't go too flat either, as it puts your calf muscles on stretch and tilts your pelvis. Don't go backless.

Flip-flops and sling-backs are a nightmare. Fit-Flops, however, are a good summer option. Birkenstocks are a bit of a fallacy too, as they are too stiff in the sole when walking; their new rubber version is much better. MBT trainers (the rocker ones with a massive sole) are appalling and would be ceremonially burnt in my office if a pair walked in. When advising on trainers, I always tell people to avoid too much cushioning and too much correction in the soles. If you have run all your life in shoes, don't join the barefoot-running craze unless you can commit to at least six months of guided and gradual conversion from an expert. Keep a golf ball under your desk to roll under your feet in socks to massage the muscles of the arches and heels. Don't shuffle when walking or walk as if you are walking on two parallel rails. Add an inch to your stride and swing your arms when walking. It activates your gluteal muscles and your core.

12. **Look out for pain-causing habits** such as vacuuming, ironing, or any activity which involves one-way twisting or holding awkward positions for any length of time.

13. **Be aware of how much extra stress you are adding to your day by unthinking use of social media.** If you can't quit it altogether, then severely curtail your use of it. Remember the old adage 'Turn on, tune in and drop out'? The app algorithms are designed by psychologists to suck you in, get you addicted, sell you stuff directly or indirectly, and crowd you with noise, most of which is inaccurate. Stop your phone distracting you by switching off the notifications. Maybe set a time once or twice a day to check your accounts and institute screen-free weekends and holidays. Manage your internal triggers for using media – when you are susceptible it is usually because you are doing something

uncomfortable; push on through. You'll be setting a good example for your children as well. And do I really need to tell you not to keep your phone by your bed? Bedrooms are for two things, sex and sleep.

14. **Confront the difficult things in life at home and work.** Awkward topics are always hard but glean the most results. Reconnect with friends and family. Don't wait for them to do come to you; life is too short. Have conversations, not arguments, with those concerned. Be vulnerable with them and they will be more honest with you. Remember, your unresolved issues come back and bite you as pain. Minimise your exposure to anyone who is bad for you.

15. **If you are a type-A perfectionist or think you can multitask, then take one, if not two, things off your to-do list daily.** Multitasking is a fallacy – it just means you don't do any of the things very well. By dealing with one task at a time, stress goes down, promptness is observed without rushing and you focus better. Also delegate more; you are not the only one who can do a good job.

16. **Reduce or eliminate dependencies such as alcohol, nicotine and even caffeine.** If you need to, lose weight. It is estimated that, for every four kilos lost, there is a resultant 17 per cent reduction in pain. That means if you have a BMI of greater than 40, you will have up to 254 per cent more pain! Losing weight is an entirely natural form of pain relief that will benefit every other aspect of your health as well. It's basically a question of calories in/calories out. Every diet ever designed simply reduces calories in some way, either through different food groups or a different eating behaviour, such as the '5:2'. With most gluten-free diets you lose weight simply because you have just cut out at least 50 per cent of the

carbohydrates in your life. Don't at any cost dump protein. If you can afford organic, go for it. Persuade your office to get a fruit bowl and get rid of any food dispensers. Nobody benefits from them.

17. **Look at your sleep**: ask yourself how high in quality it is. Do you feel recovered and fresh in the morning? Observe the following sleep hygiene rules and read a good sleep book:

- Keep the room cool and as dark as possible at night; blackout blinds are best.
- Do ten of my breaths in bed before sleep.
- Sleep on your side or back rather than on your front.
- Always get a good bed; go softer rather than harder.
- Use a supportive pillow (not down or feathers), preferably only one.
- Leave all electronics and screens out of the bedroom; get dozy in the sitting room and go to bed; don't watch TV in the bedroom.
- Don't drink coffee after 5pm.
- Limit your alcohol during the week.
- Don't lie in, get up at a regular time.

18. **Join a group.** No, not the Chronic Pain Appreciation Society – a book club, snooker or bowling team, tiddlywinks or action group. See people and connect. We are social animals and thrive off social contact. Use your social media for networking positively and look for social forums around pain; research shows they help enormously. However, you cannot beat being physically there and meeting people. Watch something funny at least once a day.

19. **Do some acts of random kindness.** These don't have to be grand gestures – just do small things often. Engage

people's eyeline and smile. On your commute, be civil and openly courteous. Help people rather than waiting for the 'fat controller' to do it – he won't! When you get your coffee you don't have to be chatty but just don't be miserable. Your behaviour matters and it changes your environment and those of others. Look good, take pride and stand tall. Remember you are someone else's scenery.

20. **And, above all, practise the breathing techniques in the previous chapter a minimum of five times a day.** It will take 15 minutes in total, maximum, and will do more than anything else to stimulate your vagus nerve and calm those fight or flight reactions that are exacerbating your aches and pains.

○ ○ ○

It is important, too, to say that this doesn't have to be a perfectionist regime that you follow rigidly for the rest of your life. Once you have got your pain and your life under control and you have seen the new place you can be in or – as Martin Luther King said, 'Once you have seen over the mountain top' – you won't want to go back to your old self.

I wish you well!

ENDNOTES

Chapter 1
1 Maté, Gabor, M.D. *When the Body Says No* 2012, Vintage Canada
2 Engel G. *The need for a new medical model: a challenge for biomedicine.* Science. 1977; 196:129–136. [PubMed]

Engel G. *The clinical application of the biopsychosocial model.* Am J Psychiatry. 1980; 137:535–544. [PubMed]

Engel GL. *How much longer must medicine's science be bounded by a seventeenth century world view?* In: White KL, ed. The Task of Medicine: Dialogue at Wickenburg. Menlo Park, Calif: The Henry Kaiser Family Foundation; 1988:113–136.
3 Loeser, JD, *Pain due to nerve injury.* Spine. 1985. 10:232-235

Loeser, J.D., *Pain and Suffering.* Clin. J. Pain 2000 16:S2-S6
4 Beecher H., *The Relationship of the significance of the wound to the pain experience.* JAMA, 1956. 161:1604-1613
5 Wall and Melzack, 1965 refs: Wall, P.D. *Pain, The Science of Suffering 1999,* London: Weidenfeld and Nicholson

Wall, P.D. and Melzack R., eds. *Textbook of Pain.* 4th Ed 1999, Churchill Livingstone: Edinburgh

Melzack, R., and P.D. Wall, T*he Challenge of Pain.* 2nd Ed. 1996. London, Penguin

Melzack, R., *Pain and Stress: A New Perspective, in Psychosocial factors in pain,* R.J. Gatchel and D.C. Turk, Editors. 1999, Guildford Press: New York
6 Benedetti, F., *Placebo Effects* 2nd Ed, Oxford University Press, 2014

Benedetti, F., *The Patient's Brain- The neuroscience behind the doctor-patient relationship.* 2011 Oxford University Press.
In relation to cultural differences in pain experienced:

Andersson, H.I., et al *Chronic pain in a geographically defined general population: Studies of differences in gender, social class, and pain localisation.* Clin J Pin, 1993. 9:174-182

Chapter 2
7 A Fayaz1, P Croft2, R M Langford3, L J Donaldson4, G T Jones5: *Prevalence of chronic pain in the UK: a systematic review and meta-analysis of population studies.* Research by The British Pain Society, 2016
8 Woolf, C.J. (2011) *Central Sensitisation: Clinical implications for the diagnosis and treatment of pain* Pain 152,3,S2-15.
9 Freeman MD, Nystrom A, Centeno C. J Brachial Plex *Chronic whiplash and central sensitization; an evaluation of the role of a myofascial trigger points in pain modulation* Peripher Nerve Inj. 2009 Apr 23;4:2. doi: 10.1186/1749-7221-4-2. .
10 Vilayanur Ramachandran TED India 2009 Ted talk "The neurons that

shaped civilization".

11 Apkarian AV1, Sosa Y, Sonty S, Levy RM, Harden RN, Parrish TB, Gitel-
man DR. *Chronic back pain is associated with decreased prefrontal and thalamic
gray matter density* J Neurosci. 2004 Nov 17;24(46):10410-5. .
12 Duhigg, C., *The Power of Habit: Why We do What We Do And How To
Change It* (Random House, 2013).
13 Maté,G., M.D. *When the Body Says No- The Cost of Hidden Stress* 2012,
Vintage Canada.

Chapter 3

14 Professor Jean M. Twenge PhD. *Why Today's Super-Connected Kids Are
Growing Up Less Rebellious, More Tolerant, Less Happy--and Completely Unprepared for Adulthood--and What That Means for the Rest of Us.* Atria Books.
2018.

   BBC Radio 4, Sept 2018: "Morality" Prof Jean Twenge interviewed by Prof
Rabbi Lord Sacks

   Tedx Talk: Prof. Jean Twenge *iGen- the Smartphone generation* 2018
15 McEwen, B., *The End of Stress as We Know It* -The Dana Press/ Joseph
Henry Press 2002
16 Sapolsky, R. M., *Why Zebras Don't Get Ulcers* 3rd Ed.2004, St.Martin's
Press, New York.
17 https://en.wikipedia.org/wiki/Da_Costa%27s_syndrome
18 Nixon PG. *The human function curve - a paradigm for our times.* Act Nerv
Super (Praha). 1982;Suppl 3(Pt 1):130-3. Nixon PGF. 1989 Hyperventilation and cardiac symptoms. Internal Medicine.10 (12), 67-84.
19 https://en.wikipedia.org/wiki/Whitehall_Study#Health_risks_associat-
ed_with_disparities_of_wealth_and_power

   https://unhealthywork.org/classic-studies/the-whitehall-study/

   North F, Syme SL, Feeney A, Head J, Shipley MJ, Marmot MG. *Explaining
socioeconomic differences in sickness absence: the Whitehall II study.* Br Med J
1993-306:361-366.

   Roberts R, Brunner EJ, White I, Marmot MG. *Gender differences in occu-
pational mobility and structure of employment in the British civil service.* Soc Sci
Med 1993;37:1415-1425.

   Stansfeld SA, Davey Smith F, Marmot MG. *Association between physi-
can and psychological morbidity in the Whitehall II study.* J Psychosom Res
1993;37:227-238.

   Marmot MG. *Social differentials in health within and between populations.*
Daedulus 1994;123:197-216.

   Marmot M. *Work and other factors influencing coronary health and sickness
absence.* Work & Stress 1994;8:191-201.
20 Cummings NA, VandenBos GR. *The twenty years Kaiser-Permanente
experience with psychotherapy and medical utilization: implications for
national health policy and national health insurance.* Health Policy Q. 1981

Summer;1(2):159-75.https://cummingsinstitute.com/wp-content/up-loads/2017/05/Collected-vol.-1-Ch-9-Twenty-Years-of-Kaiser-Experience.pdf.

21 Greg Irving, Ana Luisa Neves, Hajira Dambha-Miller et al. *International variations in primary care physician consultation time: a systematic review of 67 countries* https://bmjopen.bmj.com/content/7/10/e017902.

22 Selye, H., MD, *The Stress of Life* revised ed, 1978/84 McGraw-Hill Siang Yong Tan, MD1 and A Yip, MS2 Hans Selye (1907-1982): *Founder of the stress theory.* Singapore Med J. 2018 Apr; 59(4): 170-171 doi: 10.11622/smedj.2018043 PMCID: PMC5915631 PMID; 29748693.

23 ibid.

24 Widdowson, E.M., *Mental contentment and physical growth.* Lancet. 1951 Jun 16;1(6668):1316-8. PMID: 14842069

25 Oliver, J., *Affluenza,* 2007, Vermilion/ Random House UK

26 Phillips CJ. *The Cost and Burden of Chronic Pain* Rev Pain. 2009 Jun;3(1):2-5. doi: 10.1177/204946370090030010

A Fayaz1, P Croft2, R M Langford3, L J Donaldson4, G T Jones5 *Prevalence of chronic pain in the UK: a systematic review and meta-analysis of population studies.* BMJ Open

27 http://precedings.nature.com/documents/2561/version/1/files/npre20082561-1.pdf

https://www.wired.com/2008/01/pentagon-resear/

28 C.D. Lynch R. Sundaram J.M. Maisog A.M. Sweeney G.M. Buck Louis. *Preconception stress increases the risk of infertility: results from a couple-based prospective cohort study—the LIFE study.* Human Reproduction, Volume 29, Issue 5, 1 May 2014, Pages 1067–1075, https://doi.org/10.1093/humrep/deu032

https://www.nih.gov/news-events/news-releases/nih-study-indicates-stress-may-delay-women-getting-pregnant

29 Sarno, John E. *The Mind Body Prescription-Healing the body, Healing the pain,* 1999, Grand Central, Life and Style, Hachette Book Group

30 Mate, Gabor, M.D. *When the Body Says No* 2012, Vintage Canada

31 Plazier M1, Ost J, Stassijns G, De Ridder D, Vanneste S. *Pain characteristics in fibromyalgia: understanding the multiple dimensions of pain.* Clin Rheumatol. 2015 Apr;34(4):775-83. doi: 10.1007/s10067-014-2736-6. Epub 2014 Jul 22 https://www.medpagetoday.org/rheumatology/fibromyalgia/22431

32 https://www.cochranelibrary.com/cdsr/doi/10.1002/ 14651858. CD003348.pub3/epdf/full

---

Chapter 4

33 Maté, Gabor, M.D. "When the Body Says No" 2012, Vintage Canada

34 Prof. Pert, Candace. *Molecules of Emotion,* 1999, Touchstone Books, NY.

35 *Backache, Stress and Tension*, Hans Kraus , 2012, Skyhorse Publishing

36 Thomas CB, Greenstreet RL and V J Feletti et al., *Relationship of childhood abuse and household dysfunction to many of the leading causes of death in adults: The Adverse Childhood Experiences* (ACE) American Journal of Preventative Medicine 14, no 4 (1998) 245-58

Psychobiological characteristics in youth as predictors of five disease states: suicide, mental illness, hypertension, coronary heart disease and tumor. 1973, John Hopkins Med J

37 https://www.tandfonline.com/doi/full/10.1080/13619462.2016.1226806

38 Selye, H., MD, *The Stress of Life* revised ed., McGraw-Hill 1978/ 84

39 Sheldon Cohen, Denise Janicki-Deverts, William J. Doyle, Gregory E. Miller, Ellen Frank, Bruce S. Rabin, E and Ronald B. Turner F: *Chronic stress, glucocorticoid receptor resistance, inflammation, and disease risk.* Proc Natl Acad Sci U S A. 2012 Apr 17; 109(16): 5995–5999. Published online 2012 Apr 2. doi: 10.1073/pnas.1118355109 PMCID: PMC3341031 PMID: 22474371 Psychological and Cognitive Sciences, Psychological and Cognitive Sciences Carnegie Mellon University

40 Bullmore, Edward *The Inflamed Mind*, 2018, Short Books

41 Miller A.H.,Maletic V 2009 *Inflammation and its discontents: the role of cytokines in the pathophysiology of major depression.* Biol.Psychiatry 65 732-741

Liu Yun-Zi, Wang Yun-Xia, Jiang Chun Lei. *Inflammation: The Common Pathway of Stress-Related Diseases.* Laboratory of Stress Medicine, Faculty of Psychology and Mental Health, Second Military Medical University, Shanghai, China. Front Hum Neurosci. 2017 Jun 20;11:316. doi: 10.3389/fnhum.2017.00316. Collection 2017.

Koopman F.A., Chavan SS, Miljko S., et al. *Vagus nerve stimulation inhibits cytokine production and attenuates disease severity in rheumatoid arthritis.* Proceedings of the National Academy of Sciences. 2016; 113 8284- 8289

Groves DA, Brown VJ. *Vagal nerve stimulation: A review of its applications and potential mechanisms that mediate its clinical effects.* Neuroscience and Biobehavioural Review 2005;29;493-500

Dantzer R., Kelley K.W. *Stress and immunity: an integrated view of relationships between the brain and the immune system.* Life Sciences.1989; 44: 1995-2008

Tracey KJ. *The inflammatory reflex.* Nature. 2002 Dec 19-26;420(6917):853-9.

Nicole D. Powell, Erica K. Sloan, Michael T. Bailey, Jesusa M. G. Arevalo, Gregory E. Miller, Edith Chen, Michael S. Kobor, Brenda F. Reader, John F. Sheridan, and Steven W. Cole: *Social stress up-regulates inflammatory gene expression in the leukocyte transcriptome via ⊠-adrenergic induction of myelopoiesis* PNAS October 8, 2013 110 (41) 16574-16579; https://doi.org/10.1073/pnas.1310655110

42 Anna Hernández-Aguilera, Anna Rull et al. *Mitochondrial Dysfunction: A Basic Mechanism in Inflammation-Related Non-Communicable Diseases and Therapeutic Opportunities Mediators Inflamm.* 2013; 2013: 135698. Published online 2013 Feb 28. doi: 10.1155/2013/135698 PMCID: PMC3603328 PMID: 23533299

Hansongyi Lee,*† In Seok Lee,‡ and Ryowon Chouecor responding author*† *Obesity, Inflammation and Diet*. Pediatr Gastroenterol Hepatol Nutr. 2013 Sep; 16(3): 143–152. Published online 2013 Sep 30. doi: 10.5223/pghn.2013.16.3.143
PMCID: PMC3819692 PMID: 24224147

Mohammed S. Ellulu,1 Ismail Patimah,corresponding author2 Huzwah Khaza'ai,2 Asmah Rahmat,3 and Yehia Abed4 *Obesity and inflammation: the linking mechanism and the complications* Arch Med Sci. 2017 Jun; 13(4): 851–863. Published online 2016 Mar 31. doi: 10.5114/aoms.2016.58928
PMCID: PMC5507106 PMID: 28721154

de Mello AH1, Costa AB2, Engel JDG2, Rezin GT2. *Mitochondrial dysfunction in obesity.* Life Sci. 2018 Jan 1;192:26-32. doi: 10.1016/j.lfs.2017.11.019. Epub 2017 Nov 16.

43 Bakpro tools. www.bakpro.com This is a spinal pain release programme available online, designed by the author. It consists of a boxset of tools for patients to self- treat under guidance with an online video library to follow.

Chapter 5

44 Herald Brevik, Beverly Collett, Vittorio Ventrafridda, Rob Cohen, Derek Gallacher *Survey of chronic pain in Europe: Prevalence, impact on daily life, and treatment*, European Journal of Pain 10 (2006) also *Chronic pain epidemiology and its clinical relevance*, O. van Hecke, N. Torrance, B.H. Smith, British Journal of Anaesthesia, July 2013.

45 Tsang, A., Von Korff, M., Lee, S., Alonso, J., Karam, E., Angermeyer, M.C., et al. (2008) *Common Chronic Pain Conditions in Developed and developing Countries: Gender and age differences and comorbidity with depression-anxiety disorders.* The Journal of Pain, 9 (10), 883-891

Fillingim, R.B., King, C.D., Ribeiro-Dasilva, M.C., Rahim-Williams, B., Riley, J.L. (2009) *Sex, Gender and Pain : A review of recent clinical and experimental findings.* The Journal of Pain.10 (5).447-485

Darnall, B.D., *Sex/ gender disparity in pain and pain treatment : Closing the Gap and meeting women's treatment needs.* www.forgrace.org/images/uploads/Gender_Disparities_in_Pain_feature.pdf

Ruau,D., Liu,L., Clark,J.D., Angst,M.S., Butte, A.J., (2012) *Sex differences in reported pain across 11,000 patients captured in electronic medical records.* The Journal of Pain, 13 (3), 228-234

46 Maleki, N., Linnman, C., Borsook,D. (2012) *Brain: Her versus His migraine: multiple sex differences in brain function and structure.* DOI:10.1093/brain/aws175

47 Musgrave, D. S., Vogt, M. T., Nevitt, M. C., & Cauley, J. A. (2001). *Back problems among postmenopausal women taking estrogen replacement therapy: The Study of osteoporotic fractures*, Spine, 26 (14), 1606-1612

Fillingim R.B, Edwards R.R. (2001): *The association of hormone replacement therapy with experimental pain responses in postmenopausal women.* Pain. 2001 May; 92(1-2):229-34. PMID: 11323144

Ockene JK1, Barad DH, Cochrane BB, Larson JC, Gass M, Wassertheil-Smoller S, Manson JE, Barnabei VM, Lane DS, Brzyski RG, Rosal MC, Wylie-Rosett J, Hays J. *Symptom experience after discontinuing use of estrogen plus progestin* JAMA. (2005) July 13;294(2):183-93.

Brynhildsen JO1, Björs E, Skarsgård C, Hammar ML. *Is hormone replacement therapy a risk factor for low back pain among postmenopausal women?* Spine (Phila Pa 1976). 1998 Apr 1;23(7):809-13.

Aloisi A.M., Bachiocco V, Costantino A, Stefani R, Ceccarelli I, Bertaccini A, Meriggiola MC. *Cross-sex hormone administration changes pain in transsexual women and men.* Pain. 2007 Nov;132 Suppl 1:S60-7. Epub 2007 Mar 26.

Cervero, Fernando, *Understanding Pain* 2012, MIT Press U.S.

48 Paulson PE1, Minoshima S, Morrow TJ, Casey KL. *Gender differences in pain perception and patterns of cerebral activation during noxious heat stimulation in humans.* Pain. 1998 May;76(1-2):223-9.

Sarlani E1, Grace EG, Reynolds MA, Greenspan JD. *Sex differences in temporal summation of pain and aftersensations following repetitive noxious mechanical stimulation.* Pain. 2004 May;109(1-2):115-23.

Sarlani E1, Greenspan JD. Gender differences in temporal summation of mechanically evoked pain. Pain. 2002 May;97(1-2):163-9.

Racine M1, Tousignant-Laflamme Y, Kloda LA, Dion D, Dupuis G, Choinière M. *A systematic literature review of 10 years of research on sex/gender and experimental pain perception - part 1: are there really differences between women and men?* Pain. 2012 Mar;153(3):602-18. doi: 10.1016/j.pain.2011.11.025. Epub 2011 Dec 20.

49 Mogil, J. S. *The genetic mediation of individual differences in sensitivity to pain and its inhibition.* PNAS July 6, 1999 96 (14) 7744-7751; https://doi.org/10.1073/pnas.96.14.7744

MacGregor AJ, Andrew T, Sambrook PN, Spector TD. *Structural, psychological, and genetic influences on low back and neck pain: a study of adult female twins.* Arthritis Rheum. 2004 Apr 15;51(2):160-7.

Norbury TA1, MacGregor AJ, Urwin J, Spector TD, McMahon SB. *Heritability of responses to painful stimuli in women: a classical twin study.* Brain. 2007 Nov;130(Pt 11):3041-9. Epub 2007 Oct 11.

Nielsen CS1, Stubhaug A, Price DD, Vassend O, Czajkowski N, Harris JR. *Individual differences in pain sensitivity: genetic and environmental contributions* Pain. 2008 May;136(1-2):21-9. Epub 2007 Aug 9.

Hartvigsen J1, Nielsen J, Kyvik KO, Fejer R, Vach W, Iachine I, Leboeuf-Yde C. *Heritability of spinal pain and consequences of spinal pain: a comprehensive genetic epidemiologic analysis using a population-based sample of 15,328 twins ages 20-71 years.* Arthritis Rheum. 2009 Oct 15;61(10):1343-51. doi: 10.1002/art.24607.

Markkula R1, Järvinen P, Leino-Arjas P, Koskenvuo M, Kalso E, Kaprio J.

Clustering of symptoms associated with fibromyalgia in a Finnish Twin Cohort.
Eur J Pain. 2009 Aug;13(7):744-50. doi: 10.1016/j.ejpain.2008.09.007.
Epub 2008 Oct 19.

50 Talkington M. (2011) *Epigenetic Downregulation of GABA Signaling Perpetuates Pain.* From: https://www.painresearchforum.org/news/10272-epi-genetic-downregulation-gaba-signaling-perpetuates-pain

Zhang Z1, Cai YQ, Zou F, Bie B, Pan ZZ. *Epigenetic suppression of GAD65 expression mediates persistent pain.* Nat Med. 2011 Oct 9;17(11):1448-55. doi: 10.1038/nm.2442. https://en.wikipedia.org/wiki/NCBI_Epigenom-ics#Roadmap_Epigenomics_Project. https://www.nature.com/articles/na-ture14248[

R Yehuda et al., *Cortisol levels in Adult offspring of holocaust survivors :Relation to PTSD symptom severity in the Parent and Child* Psychoneuroendocri-nology, 27, no 1-2 (2001), 171-80

Kellermann N.P. : *Epigenetic transmission of Holocaust trauma: can nightmares be inherited?* J Psychiatry Relat Sci. 2013;50(1):33-9. https://www.theguardian.com/science/2015/aug/21/study-of-holocaust-survivors-finds-trauma-passed-on-to-childrens-genes. https://www.mail-archive.com/unponkiidoep@googlegroups.com/msg01256/gene_epigenetic_inheritance-_Holocaust_Survivor_Trauma,_GuardUK_20150821.pdf

Lipton B.H., *Nature Nurture and Human Development Journal of Prenatal and Perinatal Psychology and Health* 16, no 2 (2001) 167-80

51 Freud, Sigmund (2015) *Beyond the Pleasure Principle*, Dover Publications p.11

52 Davies, William *Nervous States,* 2018, Jonathan Cape

53 Smith, Zadie *Feel Free: Essays,* 2018, Penguin Books

54 Davies, William *Nervous States,* 2018, Jonathan Cape

55 Professor Jean M. Twenge PhD. 'iGen: Why Today's Super-Connected Kids Are Growing Up Less Rebellious, More Tolerant, Less Happy--and Completely Unprepared for Adulthood--and What That Means for the Rest of Us.' Atria Books. 2018

BBC Radio 4; 'Morality' Prof Jean Twenge interviewed by Prof Rabbi Lord Sacks

56 Simon Sinek 17 Apr 2014 "How Great Leaders Inspire Action" https://www.ted.com/talks/simon_sinek_how_great_leaders_inspire_ac-tion?language=en

57 Kahneman, Daniel *Thinking Fast and Slow* 2011 Farrar, Straus and Giroux ISBN: 9780141033570

58 Curtis, Adam 'Hypernormalisation'- Documentary BBC https://www.bbc.co.uk/programmes/p04b183c

59 Maté, Gabor, M.D. *When the Body Says No,* 2012, Vintage Canada

60 Allan Shore, *Affect Regulation and the Origin of the Self : The Neurobiology of Emotional Development* (Mahwah: Lawrence Erlbaum associates, 1994), 378.

61 Eisenberger NI1, Lieberman MD, Williams KD. *Does rejection hurt? An*

FMRI study of social exclusion. Science. 2003 Oct 10;302(5643):290-2.

Chapter 6

62 A Fayaz, P Croft, R M Langford, L J Donaldson, G.T. Jones *Prevalence of chronic pain in the UK: a systematic review and meta-analysis of population studies:* https://bmjopen.bmj.com/content/ 6/6/e010364https:// www.nice.org.uk/guidance/cg88/ documents/low-back-pain-final-scope2. https://www.britishpainsociety.org/ media-resources/

Hoy D, March L, Brooks P, et al. *The global burden of low back pain: estimates from the Global Burden of Disease 2010 study,* Annals of the Rheumatic Diseases. Published online March 24 2014

W. Brinjikji, P.H. Luetmer, B. Comstock, B.W. Bresnahan, L.E. Chen, R.A. Deyo, S. Halabi, J.A. Turner, A.L. Avins, K. James, J.T. Wald, D.F. Kallmes, and J.G. Jarvik: *Systematic Literature Review of Imaging Features of Spinal Degeneration in Asymptomatic Populations* AJNR Am J Neuroradiol. 2015 Apr; 36(4): 811–816. Published online 2014 Nov 27. doi: 10.3174/ ajnr.A4173

Masui T1, Yukawa Y, Nakamura S, Kajino G, Matsubara Y, Kato F, Ishiguro N. *Natural history of patients with lumbar disc herniation observed by magnetic resonance imaging for minimum 7 years.* J Spinal Disord Tech. 2005 Apr;18(2):121-6.

63 W. Brinjikji, P.H. Luetmer, B. Comstock, B.W. Bresnahan, L.E. Chen, R.A. Deyo, S. Halabi, J.A. Turner, A.L. Avins, K. James, J.T. Wald, D.F. Kallmes, and J.G. Jarvik. *Systematic Literature Review of Imaging Features of Spinal Degeneration in Asymptomatic Populations.* https://www.ncbi.nlm.nih. gov/pmc/articles/PMC4464797/

64 Taken from: Jakobson-Ramin, Cathryn *Crooked,* 2017 Harper Collins

65 Croft P, Macfarlane G, Papageorgiou A et al. *Outcome of low back pain in general practice: a prospective study.* BMJ 1998; 316 doi: https://doi. org/10.1136/bmj.316.7141.1356

66 A Fayaz, P Croft, R M Langford, L J Donaldson, G.T. Jones, *Prevalence of chronic pain in the UK: a systematic review and meta-analysis of population studies* https://bmjopen.bmj.com/content/6/6/e010364

67 Ekelund U, Steene-Johannessen J, Brown WJ, et al. *Does physical activity attenuate, or even eliminate, the detrimental association of sitting time with mortality? A harmonised meta-analysis of data from more than 1 million men and women.* Lancet 2016;388:1302–10.

68 Hamilton M, Healy G et al. *Too Little Exercise and Too Much Sitting: Inactivity Physiology and the Need for New Recommendations on Sedentary Behavior.* Curr Cardiovasc Risk Rep. 2008 Jul; 2(4): 292–298.

Hamilton MT, Hamilton DG, Zderic TW: *The role of low energy expenditure and sitting on obesity, metabolic syndrome, type 2 diabetes, and cardiovascular disease.* Diabetes 2007, 56:2655–2667.

69 Vertosick, Frank *Why we hurt- The natural history of pain*

Chapter 7

70 https://www.nhs.uk/conditions/fibromyalgia/

71 https://www.nice.org.uk/guidance/cg61/chapter/introduction

72 Drossman DA *Presidential address: Gastrointestinal illness and the biopsychosocial model* Psychosom Med. 1998 May-Jun;60(3):258-67.

73 Yehuda Ringel, MD, and Douglas A. Drossman, MD *Toward a Positive and Comprehensive Diagnosis of Irritable Bowel Syndrome*, University of North Carolina, Chapel Hill [Medscape Gastroenterology 2(6), 2000. © 2000 Medscape, Inc.]

Mayer EA1, Raybould HE. *Role of visceral afferent mechanisms in functional bowel disorders.* Gastroenterology. 1990 Dec;99(6):1688-704.

Emeran A. Mayer, Bruce D. Naliboff, Lin Chang, and Santosh V. Coutinho: *Stress and irritable bowel syndrome* April 2001https://doi.org/10.1152/ajpgi.2001.280.4.G519

Mayer EA1, Raybould HE. *Role of visceral afferent mechanisms in functional bowel disorders.* Gastroenterology. 1990 Dec;99(6):1688-704.

Drossman DA1, Talley NJ, Lesserman J, Olden KW, Barreiro MA. *Sexual and physical abuse and gastrointestinal illness.* Review and recommendations Ann Intern Med. 1995 Nov 15;123(10):782-94.

Lesserman J, Drossman DA, Li Z. *The reliability and validity of a sexual and physical abuse history questionnaire in female patients with gastrointestinal disorders.* Behav Med. 1995 Fall;21(3):141-50

74 Covington interview taken from: Cathryn Jakobson-Ramin, *Crooked,* 2017, Harper Collins

75 Lorimer Moseley and David Butler *Explain Pain* NOI GROUP publications

76 www.bakpro.com The one-stop-shop spinal and muscular release product and programme

---

Chapter 8

77 Lin IM and Peper E., *Psychophysiological patterns during cell phone text messaging: a preliminary study*, Applied Psychophysiol. Biofeedback, 2009

78 Dr Jacob Mendes Da Costa, 1833 -1900, civil war surgeon. Da Costa syndrome is named after him.

79 William J Kerr, Paul A Gliebe and James W Dalton, *Physical Phenomena Associated with Anxiety States: the hyperventilation syndrome* Western Journal of Medicine, 1938

80 Lum LC, *Hyperventilation: The Tip and the Iceberg*, Journal of Psychosomatic Res., 1975

Lum LC., 1987 *Hyperventilation Syndromes in Medicine and Psychiatry: A review.* Journal of The Royal Society of Medicine.229-221

81 Nixon PG. *The human function curve - a paradigm for our times.* Act Nerv Super (Praha). 1982;Suppl 3(Pt 1):130-3. https://www.researchgate.net/

figure/Human-response-to-stress-curve-according-to-Nixon-P-Practitioner-1979-Yerkes-RM_fig2_274901016

Nixon PGF. 1989 *Hyperventilation and cardiac symptoms*. Internal Medicine.10 (12), 67-84

Nixon PGF. 1993. *The Grey area of effort syndrome and hyperventilation: from Thomas Lewis to today*. Journal of the Royal College of Physicians of London 27 (4), 77-78

Cappo BM, Holmes DS. *The utility of prolonged respiratory exhalation for reducing physiological and psychological arousal in non-threatening and threatening situations*. J Psychosom Res. 1984;28(4):265-73.

Eccles R. *A role for the nasal cycle in respiratory defence*. Eur Respir J. 1996 Feb;9(2):371-6

Plum F. *Breathing is controlled independently by voluntary, emotional, and metabolically related pathways*. Arch Neurol. 1992 May;49(5):441

Meyer JS, Gotoh F. *Metabolic and electroencephalographic effects of hyperventilation. Experimental studies of brain oxygen and carbon dioxide tension, pH, EEG and blood flow during hyperventilation*. Arch Neurol. 1960 Nov;3:539-52

Hauge A, Thoresen M, Walløe L. *Changes in cerebral blood flow during hyperventilation and CO2-breathing measured transcutaneously in humans by a bidirectional, pulsed, ultrasound Doppler blood velocitymeter*. Acta Physiol Scand. 1980 Oct;110(2):167-73

Chapter 9

82 https://www.health.harvard.edu/mental-health/the-power-of-the-placebo-effect

Dr Damien G Finniss, MSc [Med] Ted J Kaptchuk Franklin Miller, PhD Prof Fabrizio Benedetti, M *Biological, clinical, and ethical advances of placebo effects* The Lancet VOLUME 375, ISSUE 9715, P686-695, FEBRUARY 20, 2010

83 https://www.hunterlab.com/blog/color-pharmaceuticals/measuring-color-generic-drugs-enhance-patient-adherence-public-safety/
https://www.sciencedaily.com/releases/2010/11/101115110959.htm

84 Pacheco, Lopez et al, 2009 Brain Behav Immun. 2010 Feb;24(2):176-85. doi: 10.1016/j.bbi.2009.08.007. Epub 2009 Aug 19.

Pacheco-López G1, Riether C et al. *Calcineurin inhibition in splenocytes induced by pavlovian conditioning*. FASEB J. 2009 Apr;23(4):1161-7. doi: 10.1096/fj.08-115683. Epub 2008 Dec 22. https://guptaprogramme.com/wp-content/uploads/2018/06/Learned-Immune-Responses-Schedlowski-Pacheco-Lopez-2010.pdf

Schedlowski M, Pacheco-López G. *The learned immune response: Pavlov and beyond.*

85 Goebel MU, Meykadeh N, Kou W, Schedlowski M, Hengge UR. *Behavioral conditioning of antihistamine effects in patients with allergic rhinitis.*

Psychother Psychosom. 2008;77(4):227-34. doi: 10.1159/000126074. Epub 2008 Apr 16.

Sabine Vits, Elvir Cesko, Paul Enck, Uwe Hillen, Dirk Schadendorf, and Manfred Schedlowski: *Behavioural conditioning as the mediator of placebo responses in the immune system.* Philos Trans R Soc Lond B Biol Sci. 2011 Jun 27; 366(1572): 1799–1807. doi: 10.1098/rstb.2010.0392

86 J. Bruce Moseley, M.D., Kimberly O'Malley, Ph.D., Nancy J. Petersen et al. *A Controlled Trial of Arthroscopic Surgery for Osteoarthritis of the Knee*: https://www.nejm.org/doi/full/10.1056/NEJMoa013259 (Moseley et al)

87 Blanchflower, David G. and Oswald, Andrew J., *Unhappiness and Pain in Modern America: a Review Essay, and Further Evidence, on Carol Graham's Happiness for All?* (November 2017). NBER Working Paper No. w24087. Available at SSRN: https://ssrn.com/abstract=3082270

88 Ted J. Kaptchuk , Elizabeth Friedlander, John M. Kelley et al. *Placebos without Deception: A Randomized Controlled Trial in Irritable Bowel Syndrome.* 2010https://doi.org/10.1371/journal.pone.0015591. https://www.youtube.com/watch?v=bbu6DolnUfM

89 Benedetti, F., 2011 *The Patient's Brain- The neuroscience behind the doctor-patient relationship.* Oxford University Press.

90 Foreman, Judy *A Nation in Pain* 2014 Oxford University Press

91 Eland, J.M., Anderson, M.J., (1977) *The Experience of pain in children. Pain: A sourcebook for nurses and other health professionals.* Boston: Little Brown and Co.

Perry,S., and Heidrich,G. (1982) Management of Pain during debridement: A survey of US burn units. PAIN, 13(3), 267-280

92 Fitzgerald,M. &Beggs,S. (2001). *The Neurobiology of pain: Developmental aspects.* The Neuroscientist, 7(3), 246-257

Fitzgerald, M., Millard C., McKintosh N., (1989) *Cutaneous hypersensitivity following peripheral tissue damage in newborn infants and its reversal with topical anaesthesia.* PAIN, 39(1), 31-36

Fitzgerald,M., Jennings, E. (1999). *The post-natal development of spinal sensory processing.* Proceedings of the National Academy of Sciences, 96(14), 7719-7722

Fitzgerald, M., Walker,S.M. (2009). *Infant pain management: A developmental neurobiological approach.* Nature Clinical Practice: Neurology, 5(1), 35-50

93 Anand, K.J.S and Hickey P.R. (1987), *Pain and its effects in the human neonate foetus.* New England Journal of Medicine,,317(21), 1323

94 Zeltzer, L.K. and Krane, E.J. (2011), *Paediatric Pain Management. In Nelson's Textbook of Paediatrics.* (19th ed.) Elsevier: New York

95 Johnston C., (2010). *From the Mouths of Babes: What have we learned from studies of pain in neonates? Paper presented to the International Association of Pain* 13th World Congress on Pain, Montreal, Canada

Barr RG1, Pantel MS, Young SN, Wright JH, Hendricks LA, Gravel R. *The response of crying newborns to sucrose: is it a "sweetness" effect?* Physiol Behav.

1999 May;66(3):409-17.

Stevens B1, Yamada J, Lee GY, Ohlsson A. *Sucrose for analgesia in newborn infants undergoing painful procedures.* Cochrane Database Syst Rev. 2013 Jan 31;(1):CD001069. doi: 10.1002/14651858.CD001069.pub4

Akman I1, Ozek E, Bilgen H, Ozdogan T, Cebeci D. *Sweet solutions and pacifiers for pain relief in newborn infants.* J Pain. 2002 Jun;3(3):199-202.

Slater R1, Cornelissen L, Fabrizi L, Patten D, Yoxen J, Worley A, Boyd S, Meek J, Fitzgerald M. *Oral sucrose as an analgesic drug for procedural pain in newborn infants: a randomised controlled trial.* Lancet. 2010 Oct 9;376(9748):1225-32. doi: 10.1016/S0140-6736(10)61303-7.

96 Achor, Shaun www.goodthinkinc.com

97 Harari, Y.N. "Sapiens" 2014 Harvill Secker

98 https://en.wikipedia.org/wiki/B._F._Skinner

99 Williams, James. *Stand out of our Light: Freedom and Resistance in the Attention Economy* ISBN 9781108429092 Oxford. https://blogs.lse.ac.uk/lsereviewofbooks/2018/06/18/lse-feature-interview-with-nine-dots-prize-winner-james-williams-on-new-book-stand-out-of-our-light-freedom-and-resistance-in-the-attention-economy/

BIBLIOGRAPHY

William C Dement, *The Promise of Sleep,* 2000, Dell

Benedetti, F., *Placebo Effects,* 2nd Ed, Oxford University Press, 2014

Benedetti, F., 2011 *The Patient's Brain – The Neuroscience behind the Doctor-Patient Relationship*, Oxford University Press.

Boddice, R. *Pain-A Very Short Introduction,* 2017, Oxford University Press

Bourke, J., *The Story of Pain,* 2014, Oxford University Press

Bullmore, Edward *The Inflamed Mind,* 2018, Short Books

Cady, Melissa *Paindemic,* 2016, Morgan James Publishing

Cervero, Ferdnando, *Understanding Pain,* 2012, MIT Press U.S.

Davies, William *Nervous States,* 2018, Jonathan Cape

Duhigg, Charles, *The Power of Habit,* 2013, Random House Books

Foreman, Judy *A Nation in Pain,* 2014, Oxford University Press

Haines, Steve, *Pain is Really Strange,* 2015, Singing Dragon

Haines, Steve, *Anxiety is Really Strange,* 2018, Singing Dragon

Harari, Y.N. *Sapiens,* 2014, Harvill Secker

Harari, Y.N. *21 Lessons for the 21st Century,* 2018, Penguin Random House

Hardy, Benjamin *Willpower Doesn't Work,* 2018, Hachette Books

Hari, Jonathan *Lost Connections,* 2018, Bloomsbury Circus

Huffington, Arianna, *The Sleep Revolution,* 2016, Penguin

James, Oliver *Affluenza,* 2007, Vermilion/ Random House UK

Jakobson-Ramin, Cathryn *Crooked,* 2017, Harper Collins

Kahneman, Daniel *Thinking Fast and Slow,* 2011, Farrar, Straus and Giroux

Lewis, C.S., *The Problem of Pain,* 2015, Harper Collins

Martin, Paul *The Sickening Mind Brain, Behaviour, Immunity and Disease,* 2005, Harper Perennial

Mate, Gabor, M.D. *When the Body Says No,* 2012, Vintage Canada

McEwen, Bruce *The End of Stress as We Know It,* 2002, Joseph Henry Press

Meadows, Guy, *The Sleep Book,* 2014, Orion

Wallace B Mendelson MD, The Science of Sleep, 2014, Ivy Press

Moseley, Lorimer and Butler, David *Explain Pain*, 2015, NOI Group publications

Moseley, Lorimer and Butler, David *Explain Pain Supercharged,* 2017, NOI Group publications

Nelson, Douglas *The Mystery of Pain,* 2013, Singing Dragon / Jessica Kingsley Publishing

O'Mahony, Seamus *Can Medicine be Cured?,* 2019, Head of Zeus

O'Sullivan, S., *It's all in your Head,* 2015, Chatto and Windus, Penguin Random House

Ramachandran V.S. *The Tell-Tale Brain,* 2011, William Heinemann

Sapolski, Robert M. *Why Zebras Don't Get Ulcers* 3rd ed., 2004, St Martin's Griffin

Sarno, John E. *The Mind Body Prescription-Healing the body, Healing the Pain*, 1999, Grand Central.

Sarno, John E., *The Divided Mind*, 2009, Duckworth Overlook

Selye, Hans *The Stress of Life* rev. ed., 1978, McGraw -Hill

Smith, Zadie *Feel Free: Essays*, 2018, Penguin Books

Twenge, Professor Jean M. *iGen: Why Today's Super-Connected Kids Are Growing Up Less Rebellious, More Tolerant, Less Happy and Completely Unprepared for Adulthood and What That Means for the Rest of Us*, 2018, Atria Books

Van der Kolk, Bessel, *The Body Keeps the Score*, 2015, Penguin

Vertosick, Frank *Why We Hurt – The Natural History of Pain*, 2005, Harvest Books

Walker, Matthew, *Why We Sleep,* ,2017, Allen Lane

Wall, P. *Pain: The Science of Suffering*, 2000, Columbia University Press

ACKNOWLEDGEMENTS

I have found it very difficult to decide who to thank first for helping me to write this book.

I would of course be nowhere on my journey without all of my patients of the last 27 years. Without their trust I would have learned nothing and, with their continuing loyalty, I am still learning to adapt what I do in clinical practice. I cherish the many conversations and debates we have had along the way, not all of them easy but most of them happy and uplifting. Everyday, they bring me a new challenge and a desire to move forward in the fight to relieve pain in all its guises.

On a personal note, I must thank my noble, long-suffering wife Bex, who encouraged me to embark on this book and realise a small dream. She has tirelessly supported me in all my moods and the long hours of writing, whilst trying to run a busy practice. She has been my most rigorous critic and my most devoted supporter. Thank you, too, to my two wonderful children whom I adore in equal measure.

I owe much to my family 'the Potter clan' and my parents' enduring love and support.

I am immensely grateful to Catherine Gibbs at Short Books who first persuaded me to write down my thoughts on pain and for handing me over to Aurea Carpenter who has deftly and succinctly managed me through the process of authorship. I remember fondly our first lunch together, at which the Short Books team grilled and roasted me intellectually and sent me packing with nine chapters to write. Thank you all.

Thanks also to Caroline Wood, my agent at Felicity Bryan, who has always been on hand to manage my doubts and beliefs as well as advise me technically.

Lindsay Nicholson has patiently advised me not to make perfection the enemy of the good and has kept me on point throughout. I could not have done it without her.

I want to thank, for many reasons, Alan Howard. He has supported and facilitated many ideas I have had over the past few years and I owe him much. Thank you friend.

Dame Gail Rebuck has always supported me with advice in my practice life and has encouraged me throughout the writing of this book. I am truly grateful.

Finally, I owe a debt of gratitude to all of my professional colleagues, who have shared their wisdom and with whom I have worked both here and abroad. They have taught me to be always curious, to 'kick the tyres' of what we know and occasionally reach a little beyond our grasp.

Thank you all.

INDEX

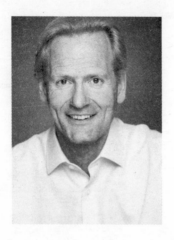

NICK POTTER is a registered osteopath who specialises in cervical spine injuries as well as head, neck and facial pain syndromes. Since qualifying in 1993, he has split his time between his clinical practice and performance medicine. He has worked with elite track athletes, professional golfers, tennis players and Formula 1 drivers. He is a keen and active lecturer and has travelled all over the world to teach, as well as treat, patients. Over the last 15 years he has highlighted and elucidated the concept of the upper cervical syndrome' for which he has formulated treatment techniques with great success. He has also been consultant to a lading hedgefund on human performance and wellbeing for 6 years. He fundamentally believes in making treatment fun and as easy as possible, whenever possible, and cannot see what could be more interesting than people. Perhaps most important of all for patients, he has had a spinal injury himself.